LORRAINE KELLY'S
JUNK-FREE
CHILDREN'S
EATING PLAN

WITH CARINA NORRIS

Virgin BOOKS

First published in Great Britain in 2007 by
Virgin Books Ltd
Thames Wharf Studios
Rainville Road
London
W6 9HA

Copyright © Lorraine Kelly 2007
Written with Carina Norris

Images: pages 10, 13, 14, 32, 54, 61, 67, 88, 101, 103 copyright © Shutterstock, Inc. 2006;
pages 53, 60, 102, 122, 124 copyright © Corbis;
page 8 copyright © iStockphoto.

A catalogue record for this book is available from the British Library.

ISBN 978 0 7535 1129 9

The paper used in this book is a natural, recyclable product made from wood grown in sustainable
forests. The manufacturing process conforms to the regulations of the country of origin.

Designed by seagulls.net

Printed and bound in Italy

CONTENTS

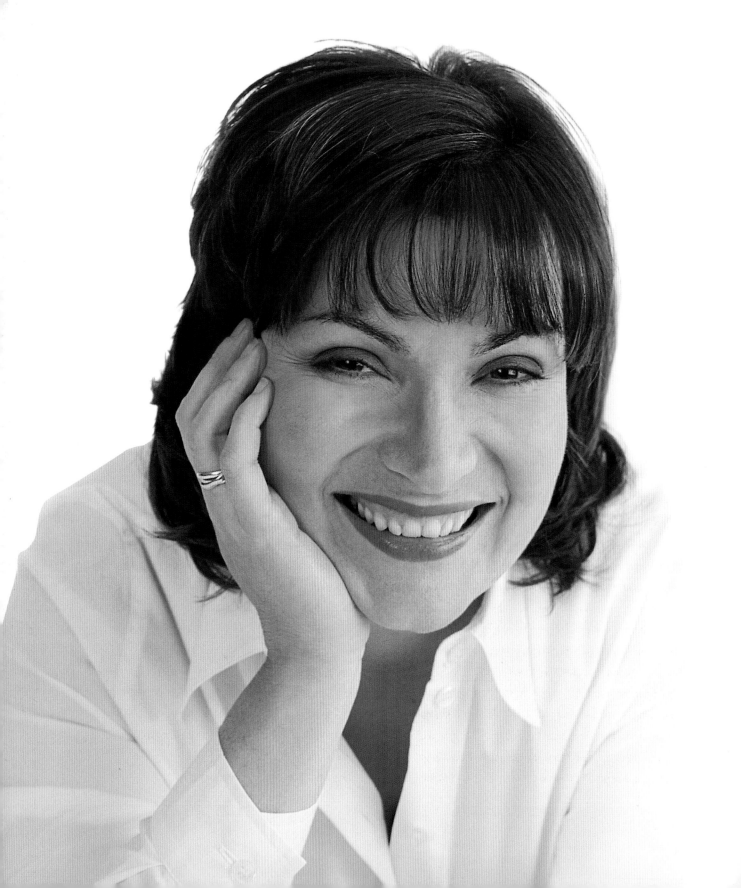

INTRODUCTION

I'm a mum and I know how tough it can be to get your children to eat well, but more than ever before it is vitally important to make sure our kids are eating healthy meals and getting some exercise.

With this country on the brink of an obesity epidemic it is clear that we need to do something to stop our children turning into a nation of couch potatoes.

I feel very strongly that all of us who are lucky enough to have kids need to make an effort to ensure that the food that goes into their mouths is going to be good for them at least most of the time. I want to show you how to help your child to eat healthily without turning into a 'food freak' and without banning the foods that kids love to eat.

I happen to think that there is nothing wrong with pizzas, burgers, chicken nuggets and sweeties if you have them now and again. But no child should be living on a diet of sugary drinks and fast food. The danger is they will get fat, unhealthy, unhappy and they are more likely to develop heart disease and diabetes. It's an appalling thought, but a bad diet may also cut years off their lives.

But do not despair. There are lots of things you can do to keep your child fit and well. You don't need to be a professional cook and it won't cost a fortune. In fact, if you cut down on those take-aways and ready meals you will end up saving money, and a few sensible changes in what you serve up to them will make all the difference.

This book is packed full of common sense information and ideas and is all about making your life easier. If your kids are eating well they will have more energy, they will do better at school, their skin and hair will improve and so will their behaviour.

And what parent wouldn't want that?

HOW THIS BOOK WORKS

In this book you'll learn how to 'de-junk' and improve your child's diet – and your whole family's as well – so at the end of the 6-Week Junk-Free Plan you'll all be eating a healthy, balanced diet, and enjoying it!

This doesn't mean you'll never be able to go out together as a family and enjoy eating at a fast-food restaurant. It just shouldn't be your *only* option when you're away from home. And chocolate and sweets won't be banned – they're just saved for occasional treats. If you totally cut out children's favourite treats and foods, they'll be miserable, and they'll rebel. And no parent wants that!

If you remove the less healthy foods from a child's diet, you have to replace them with something better. But most of us don't have time to prepare complicated recipes, and budget is always a concern when trying to feed a family. I know from experience that children can be stubborn and picky, and you don't want to buy strange, unfamiliar ingredients your family may turn their noses up at.

So, you'll find that this plan is practical and simple. There are loads of ideas and tips for quick and healthy meals, which won't have you tied to the kitchen for hours on end. The last thing you want at the end of a hectic day is to spend hours fussing around in the kitchen, chopping endless vegetables and creating a horrible mountain of washing-up. So, my philosophy is: if a meal can't be on the table in less than half an hour, then forget about it (at least until one of those rare occasions when you actually have some time on your hands).

With this plan you'll all be eating plenty of tasty food – including many favourites such as chips, pizzas and chicken nuggets. They've just been made healthier, without losing any of the taste or kid-appeal. And your children will still be able to enjoy treats and snacks – in fact, they're vital for the plan. It's all about enjoying food!

The key to this plan is that it allows your children plenty of choice, but within limits of course. Behind the scenes, you're in charge, but it gets them involved in food and its preparation, so they learn that healthy eating is interesting – and fun! And because the plan is based on sound nutritional science your child will obtain all the nutrients they need to grow up strong, fit and healthy.

These days, more than ever, we need to make sure that our children are getting a good well-balanced, healthy diet. Our children are simply eating far too much rubbish and they aren't exercising as much as they should, preferring to spend their time in front of the computer playing games or emailing their friends.

In **Part 1**, **Chapter 1**, you'll find out about what junk food is and why many modern children's diets differ from what they should be.

Chapters 2 and 3 will show you why it's important for children to eat healthily, and how what they eat now can affect their health when they grow up. This is also where you learn where to find all the nutrients your children need, with useful tips and ideas for persuading children to eat them – and we all know how difficult that can be!

In **Chapter 4**, we'll introduce the link between food, mood and behaviour, and explain how good nutrition can help keep children calm and improve their performance in school.

Good food also boosts the immune system, so we'll be telling you how a healthy diet can help prevent children from picking up every germ that's going around.

But all the healthy food in the world isn't a scrap of use if your child won't eat it, so **Chapter 5** is all about persuading children to eat a nutritious diet. Children know what they like, and all too often it's not what they should be eating. If you try to force them to eat something they don't want, they'll dig their little heels in all the harder! So we've come up with plenty of clever ways to convince your child that healthy eating is tasty and fun!

Part 2 is the 6-Week Junk-Free Eating Plan – how to actually revamp your child's diet, and your whole family's as well. Each week, you'll sort out one part of your 'foodie life' – starting with your store cupboard and your shopping habits, and working through breakfast, lunch, dinner and snacks. Once you've completed the 6-Week Junk-Free Plan, you'll be eating a healthy diet, and you'll already be feeling the benefits!

But this isn't the end – it's only the beginning. **Part 3** will show you how to maintain your new healthy lifestyle – while allowing you the little indulgences that make life that extra bit nicer. If you eat healthily almost all of the time, you're allowed to relax sometimes. Even a junk-free family can enjoy an occasional meal in a fast-food restaurant, and a child should be able to 'splurge' at a friend's party without feeling guilty.

We'll show you how to adapt the 6-Week Junk-Free Plan for children who need to lose weight. Childhood obesity is often in the news – it's a big problem, and it's important to tackle it. So we'll show you how this can be done. You can also adapt the plan for older and younger children, vegetarians, sporty children and children with food allergies and intolerances. We'll explain how to tweak your favourite recipes to make them healthier, and give you plenty of tips and advice to stop your healthy intentions from flying out of the window when you're out and about.

It is a sad fact that if you asked some children where milk came from they'd say, 'From a carton' or 'From the supermarket'. We need our children to be enthusiastic and inquisitive about food. We all know what little 'sponges' children can be, anxious to soak up knowledge, so it's up to us to feed their little minds as well as their faces. Tell them where foods come from, let them help in the kitchen, let them grow a few vegetables – even if it's only some cress seeds on a piece of kitchen towel. This book has heaps of different ways to share your enthusiasm for healthy eating with your little ones.

Exercise is important too – as important as healthy eating is, it needs to be fitted into an all-round healthy lifestyle. So in **Part 4** we have plenty of fun advice on getting your family more active.

Finally, in **Part 5**, we've got the recipes. Plenty of the meals in the 6-Week Junk-Free Plan are very simple ideas with just a few ingredients – so they don't need recipes. But, if more explanation is needed, you'll see the 📖 symbol, and you can turn to the back of the book for full instructions, and helpful symbols to show you the nutrients each recipe is especially rich in. There's nothing complicated or time consuming in this book. All the recipes are made with easy-to-find and inexpensive ingredients.

So dive in, de-junk, and enjoy.

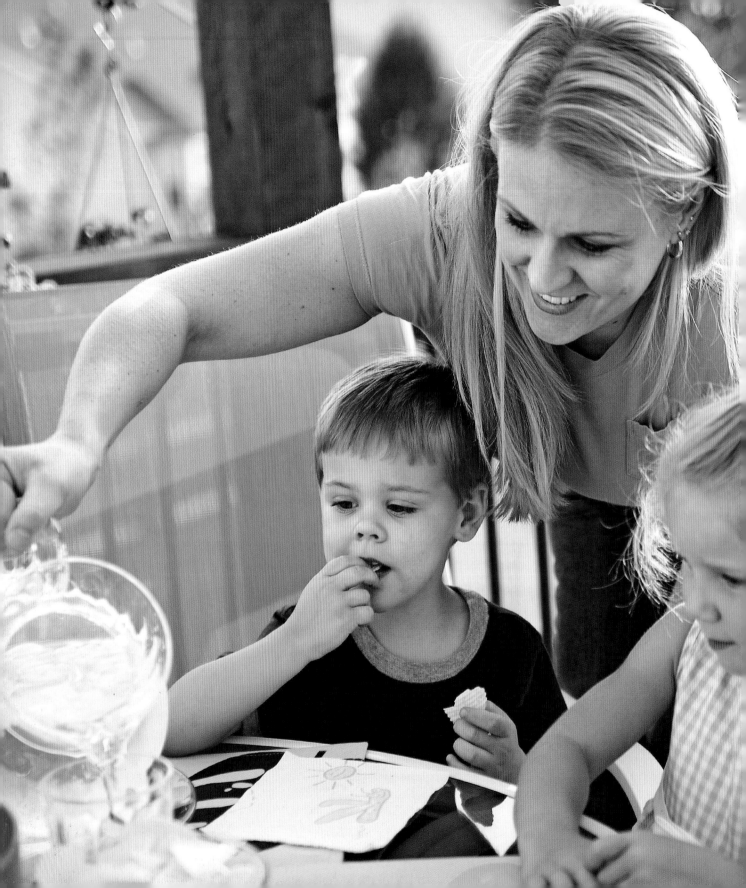

PART 1
YOUR
CHILD'S
DIET

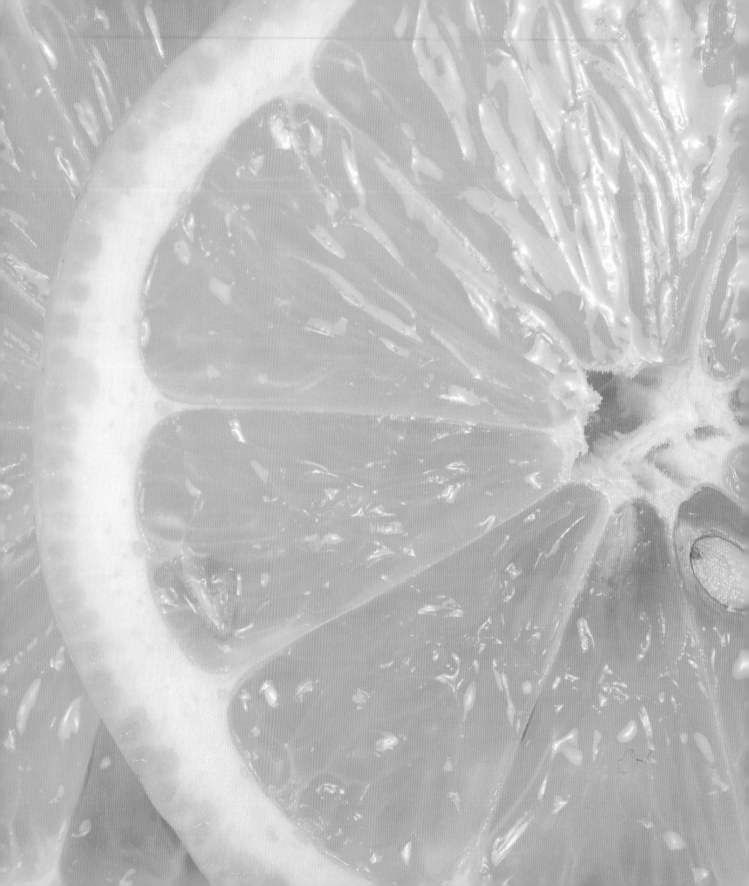

CHAPTER ONE
WHAT IS 'JUNK FOOD'?

We all have a picture in our minds of what junk food is. The word 'junk' conjures up images of greasy burgers and chips, or crisps and sugary doughnuts. But what do junk foods have in common?

The *Concise Oxford Dictionary* defines junk food as 'food with little nutritional value', but there's actually more to the story than that. Let's take a beefburger and chips for example – most people would say this is classic junk food. But it has plenty of nutritional value if you look at it in a certain way – the beef is a rich source of protein and iron, and the potatoes the chips are made from are a nutritious food. Therefore, our burger and chips are 'good and nutritious', and certainly not junk – or so the manufacturer would have us believe ...

But wait a minute – the beefburger could be full of fat, particularly harmful saturated fat. The potato will most likely be deep fried, bumping up the fat content even more. And chips are generally served with plenty of salt – another unhealthy addition.

So, although our burger and chips *do* contain some 'good' nutrients, they're also high in harmful ones. And it's the *balance* of good and bad nutrients that makes a food 'junk' or healthy.

Here's another example: nuts are high in fat. Ninety per cent of the calories in a Brazil nut come from fat. So does this make nuts 'junk food'? Definitely not! The fat in nuts is 'healthy' fat, the unsaturated kind that in moderate amounts decreases our risk of heart disease. Provided they don't eat so many that their calorie intake goes sky high, and so long as the nuts are plain (not salted), and, obviously, assuming that your little one has no dangerous nut allergies, nuts are a great addition to a child's diet.

Sadly, many of the foods children eat today are high in harmful saturated fat, sugar and salt, and, when eaten regularly, can also lead to overweight and obesity, with all the associated health problems. Many children's diets are also low in healthy fruit, vegetables and fibre. And this combination is what we mean by a 'junk food diet'.

why is eating healthily important?

A poor diet can have many effects on a child, but a good diet helps them to fulfil their potential, giving them:

- Strong immunity, to help prevent them from picking up every cough and cold that's going around.
- Better concentration, so that they can work hard at school.
- Plenty of energy, for play and sports.
- Smooth skin, glossy hair and healthy nails, so that their confidence blossoms.
- Decreased risk of asthma, and helping to prevent existing asthma from worsening.
- The best resources to grow healthy and strong – at its worst, poor nutrition can affect a child's growth.

Children with unhealthy diets are likely to be less healthy when they grow up. It's a scary thought, but doctors have found conditions once seen as diseases of middle age, such as high blood pressure, high cholesterol levels, clogged arteries and type 2 diabetes, in primary-school-age children.

But it's not all doom and gloom. By feeding your children a healthy diet, you can give them the best possible start in life, and set the stage for a long and healthy adulthood. Becoming a mum was the best thing that ever happened to me, but the responsibility is sometimes overwhelming. We're the ones who need to do our best to make our kids grow up happy and healthy.

Children who learn to enjoy healthy foods when they are young are more likely to choose them in the future. Our food preferences are almost totally learned – we're not born with an aversion to cabbage but we may be put off it for life if we associate it with a soggy mound of overcooked sludge. But if your child enjoys vegetables, thinks wholemeal bread is tastier than white and is used to grabbing an apple as a snack, they'll be more likely to do the same later, when they're older and buying their own food. The wider the range of healthy food you can offer them as children the more you will be helping them to develop their tastes and appreciation of good food. And be prepared for some surprises as you begin to introduce new foods. You may personally hate olives, but discover that your eight-year-old thinks they're really cool!

what is a 'poor diet'?

It sounds a bit of a contradiction, but many of today's children are suffering from overnutrition and undernutrition at the same time.

OVERNUTRITION

Some children eat more than they need (especially the unhealthy foods) with the inevitable result that they put on weight. And by eating too much saturated fat they increase their risk of heart disease in the future.

UNDERNUTRITION

Many of the foods children eat are high in calories, fat and sugar, but low in nutrients such as vitamins and minerals. At the same time, many children don't eat enough fruit, vegetables and 'wholefoods', which means that they're missing out on vital nutrients.

In the most recent official National Diet and Nutrition Survey of children's nutrition, children were found to be eating too much of the things they shouldn't, and not getting enough of the nutrients they should. So, you can see that it's quite possible to be overweight, and still suffer from a nutritional deficiency.

The answer? Fill children up with tasty healthy foods, so they won't want the less nutritious so-called 'junk foods'.

It's not rocket science. You just need a basic understanding of the nutrients children need, to know the foods they're found in — and plenty of ingenious tips and tricks to get them to eat them! You need to make the healthy foods as tasty and appealing as the unhealthy ones. You think you couldn't make a burger that beats the ones at your child's favourite fast-food restaurant? You could! That's where this book comes in, so read on ...

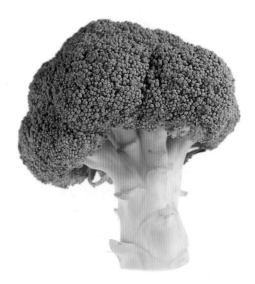

CHAPTER TWO

NUTRITION FOR CHILDREN

Childhood – it's hard to think of a stage in our lives when it's more important to eat healthily. Because children are growing and developing, it's vital for them to have a balanced diet, with all the nutritional building blocks for a healthy body.

Now it's time for the science bit! You don't need to understand all of it, and you certainly don't need to learn all of it. But having a grasp of the nutrients that children need, and knowing *why* you're making changes to your family's diet, can help everything slot into place.

If you like, just skim through the next section about protein, carbohydrates, fats, vitamins and the like, and go on to the part about foods for children – it's full of useful information and tips on how to get your children to eat the food that's good for them. And you'll find all the practical

advice you need in the 6-Week Junk-Free Plan and later in the book.

You don't need to panic if it doesn't look as if your child's diet ticks all the boxes for every single nutrient they need every day. Although it's best to keep children regularly topped up with all the different nutrients, a few days when your child's healthy diet takes a nosedive, because life suddenly goes pear-shaped or they go through a phase of turning up their nose at everything you put in front of them, won't harm them in the long run.

What children need

energy (calories)

Nowadays, in our diet-conscious society, you might be forgiven for thinking that calories are the enemy, but it's important not to think of calories as 'bad'. Calories (kcal) are simply energy, which all of us need, especially children. We need energy to move about, grow, digest our food, keep warm and think – in fact, to stay alive. Calories only become a 'problem' when we eat more than we need, and the excess is stored as fat.

Children need proportionally more energy (for their size) than adults, because they're generally more active. Childhood growth also requires extra calories. And children need proportionally more protein, vitamins and minerals, because they're still developing.

Unfortunately, many foods are high in calories but low in nutrients. We call the worst of these foods 'empty calories' – in other words, they contain calories, but little or no other nutritional benefit. If children eat too many of these kinds of foods, they'll reach their recommended calorie intake before they meet their nutritional targets. It's no surprise to learn that these high-calorie, low-nutrient foods are those we call 'junk food'.

What children need is food that is 'nutrient dense' – packed with nutrients. These are the foods we're going to be concentrating on in the 6-Week Junk-Free Plan.

When all is said and done, we don't want to get bogged down with calories – and this book isn't about calorie counting. Calories are useful for comparisons – seeing the way that children need more energy at certain ages, and to help you decide between different brands of food in the supermarket, for example. But that's it. If you and your child eat a healthy, balanced diet, you won't need to worry about counting calories – life's too short for that! And we certainly don't want our children to be thinking about calories.

CALORIES FOR AGES AND STAGES

	Boys/Men	Girls/Women
Children		
7–10 years	1,970	1,740
11–14 years	2,200	1,845
15–18 years	2,755	2,110
Adults		
19–59 years	2,550	1,920
60–74 years	2,355	1,900
75 +	2,100	1,810

These are the Estimated Average Requirements for children (and adults, for comparison). But it's important to remember that all children are different – there's no such thing as an 'average' child!

the building blocks

The main nutrients children need are the so-called macronutrients. These are needed in relatively large quantities:

▸▸ Protein
▸▸ Carbohydrates
▸▸ Fats

Although they're not strictly nutrients, children also need:

▶▶ Fibre

▶▶ Water

Then there are the micronutrients – they're called 'micro' because they're only needed in minuscule quantities, but it's important not to forget about them. Micronutrients are responsible for many of the chemical reactions that keep our bodies running smoothly, and include:

▶▶ Vitamins

▶▶ Minerals

▶▶ Phytochemicals (plant chemicals)

Protein

It's vital for children to get enough protein, for growth, and for essential maintenance of their bodies.

Children have proportionally higher protein needs than adults and they also need extra protein at certain times, such as when they're going through a growth spurt, or when they're recovering from an illness or injury.

Fortunately, most children in the UK get plenty of protein. What we need to ensure is that it comes from healthy sources that are low in unhealthy fat and salt.

Choose protein that's as near as possible to its natural, unprocessed state. That means buying good-quality lean meat, chicken and fish, rather than sausages, burgers, and other processed or 're-formed' meat products, which generally contain much more fat and salt, as well as bulkers, fillers and water, to make them go further. By making simple, tasty meals from scratch, using natural ingredients, not only will you slash the fat and salt content of your children's diets, but you'll also know exactly what goes into their food, which is very reassuring.

How much protein?

These are the estimated average requirements for children, in grams per day.

	Boys	Girls
7–10 years	23g	23g
11–14 years	34g	33g

Good sources of protein include:

Animal sources:

▶▶ Lean meat

▶▶ Poultry

▶▶ Fish

▶▶ Eggs

▶▶ Dairy products (eg milk, cheese (including cottage cheese) and yoghurt)

Non-animal sources:

▶▶ Pulses (beans and lentils)

▶▶ Nuts (eg almonds, Brazil nuts, hazelnuts, cashew nuts)

▶▶ Seeds (eg sunflower, sesame, pumpkin)

▶▶ Quorn, and soya products such as tofu and soya meat substitutes

▶▶ Wholegrains also contain a small amount of protein

Both animal and non-animal protein sources have their own advantages and disadvantages. Animal protein is a concentrated protein source, which is easiest for the body to use, but it contains saturated fat, which we should minimise in our children's diets. Vegetarian protein sources are less easy for the body to use, but they lack the bad saturated fat, and also contain healthy unsaturated fats. They also contain fibre, which is good for digestion, and heart healthy too.

Probably the healthiest option is for children to get their protein from as wide a variety of protein sources as possible.

Carbohydrates

Carbohydrates are one of the body's main fuels, so they're very important for children.

Carbohydrates can be divided into:

▶▶ Starches

▶▶ Sugars

▶▶ Fibre

Starch

Starches are basically lots of sugar units stuck together, which is why they're also called 'complex carbohydrates'. Ultimately, the body is powered by a simple sugar unit called glucose, but it doesn't need its energy supply in 'neat sugar' form.

The body much prefers to break down starches to their component sugars, producing a more gradual, 'slow-release' supply of energy, which is far less of a stress to the system.

So, we know that carbohydrates are the main fuel for children, and that starches are the healthiest carbohydrates. This is because they produce 'slow fuel'.

SLOW-FUEL FOODS

- **Oats (eg porridge and oatcakes, but not instant oats)**
- **Muesli (no added sugar)**
- **Chick peas and kidney beans**
- **Lentils**
- **Wholemeal bread**
- **Fresh fruit (especially apples, oranges, kiwifruit, berries and cherries, but not dried fruit such as raisins)**
- **Nuts and seeds**

When your child eats a sugary food, the sugar is quickly digested and absorbed, and their blood sugar level shoots up, providing a quick energy buzz. But the energy is all too quickly used up, leaving the child hungry and tired, and wanting more food – usually another sugar boost.

When a child eats a starchy food, it's digested more slowly and absorbed more gradually, as it takes time to break the complex starch down into simple sugars. The child's blood sugar level rises more slowly, and is maintained for longer, keeping them sustained for longer, and avoiding the sudden fall in blood sugar and resulting 'sugar low'.

Wholegrains: The starches that provide the most sustained energy source for children are wholegrains – things like brown pasta, wholemeal bread and brown rice. This is because they are the slowest to digest and absorb.

Also, wholegrains are more nutritious. Because they're less processed than refined, 'white' starchy carbohydrates, they contain more 'goodness'. They retain more of the important nutrients, such as the B vitamins and vitamin E, and the minerals magnesium and zinc. (Non-wholemeal white flour, however, is fortified with calcium and folic acid.)

You might think that all this makes wholemeal carbs the obvious best choice for children – after all, we want to keep them sustained between meals so that they don't get hungry or want to grab a fatty or sugary snack. And we've already said that children need plenty of vitamins and minerals. But wholegrains are also high in fibre. Now, while fibre is a vital part of anyone's diet, and most children don't eat enough of it, it is so good at filling children up it can lead to them becoming full before they've eaten enough to

OTHER CARBOHYDRATES

There's more to carbs than bread, rice and pasta. You can ring the changes with other healthy grains such as:

- Couscous
- Bulgur wheat
- Barley
- Oats
- Buckwheat

If your child turns up his or her nose at unfamiliar grains, don't give up at the first attempt. Porridge and homemade muesli (see the Recipes Section in Part 5) are simple enough for children to make, or help with, which always makes things more fun. And couscous can be coloured prettily with spices such as turmeric. Barley can be slipped into soups, and buckwheat can be gently toasted before cooking to make its little pyramid-shaped grains even tastier.

receive all the nutrients they need. If you have a strapping 14-year-old boy, he'll probably have a healthy enough appetite to eat 'wholemeal everything' – and he'll benefit from it. But if you have, say, a six-year-old with a picky appetite, see if she complains of being unable to finish her meals when they're high in wholegrains. If this is the case, it's best for her to have some less filling, white bread, rice or pasta, until she's older and bigger, and her appetite grows too. You could also try the 'half-and-half' semi-wholemeal breads and pastas that are available.

Sugar

Children love sugar – and most eat too much of it. The official recommendation is for no more than 11–12 teaspoons of sugar per day for primary-school-aged children. But the most recent government survey of children's diets found that children eat an average of $17\frac{1}{2}$ teaspoons of sugar each day. And it's easy to see why with the huge variety of high-sugar foods that are targeted at children, and when you consider the amount of 'hidden sugars' that sneak into everyday foods.

RECOMMENDED MAXIMUM INTAKES OF SUGAR – LESS IS BETTER:

	Boys	Girls
7–10 years	$12\frac{1}{2}$ teaspoons	11 teaspoons
11–14 years	$13\frac{1}{2}$ teaspoons	$11\frac{1}{2}$ teaspoons

▶▶ Sugar, especially eaten between meals, can contribute to tooth decay.

▶▶ Sweets are often described as 'empty calories' because they supply calories but little or no nutritional benefit – just a nice taste!

▶▶ Sugary snacks are also often high in fat – think of chocolate, ice cream, biscuits and cakes.

▶▶ Because they taste so good, and don't keep children feeling full for long, all too often sugary treats crowd out more nutritious foods from children's diets.

But there's no such thing as a totally 'bad' food – and sugars are no exception. It's a question of how much, how often and the kinds of sugars our children have.

Unfortunately, it's hard to figure out just how much of the sweet stuff our children eat, because a lot is hidden in processed foods, like cakes, bars and biscuits, breakfast cereals (even the non-sugar-coated ones) and tinned fruit. You'll also find a surprising amount lurking in savoury foods, such as tinned spaghetti, baked beans and vegetables, and tomato ketchup and other table sauces.

The secret is to learn the many names manufacturers use for sugars (you'll notice that many end in '*ose*') and look out for them on the labels – the nearer they are to the beginning of the ingredients list, the more of that sugar the food contains. Armed with this knowledge, you can choose the low-sugar options.

Look out for:

▶▶ Sucrose
▶▶ Fructose
▶▶ Glucose
▶▶ Lactose
▶▶ Maltose
▶▶ Dextrose
▶▶ Treacle
▶▶ Honey
▶▶ Golden syrup
▶▶ Corn syrup
▶▶ Maple syrup
▶▶ Invert sugar
▶▶ Raw sugar
▶▶ Hydrolysed starch

If a label says:

Sugar free – it means the product is free of natural sugars but may well contain artificial sweeteners.

Low sugar – it contains less than 5g sugar per 100g of the product, but it could often also contain artificial sweeteners.
No added sugar – it has had no natural sugars added but could contain fruit juice concentrate, honey or artificial sweeteners.

Artificial sweeteners: Scientists are still not 100% sure of the safety of artificial sweeteners, particularly in children, and sweeteners also encourage children to develop a sweet tooth.

Many processed foods contain artificial sweeteners and so are best avoided where possible. You'll commonly find them in ice lollies, yoghurts and desserts, ice cream, flavoured crisps, sauces, cakes, biscuits and ready meals. If you don't want to feed your children these chemicals, keep your eyes open for them on the labels. You'll find plenty of products without them. Examples of artificial sweeteners include aspartame, sorbitol, saccharine and acesulphame K.

HOMEMADE FIZZ

My friend's little boy is adorable but give him some fizzy drink and he's running around the house like a little maniac. Here is a simple recipe for a refreshing alternative to unhealthy fizzy drinks – it contains no added sugar or sweeteners. For a non-fizzy drink, use still water.

For a long cold drink:
⅓ fresh fruit juice
⅔ sparkling water
A slice of orange
A couple of ice cubes

Natural sweeteners: 'Natural' sweeteners such as honey and molasses are still 'sugars', and still cause a rapid rise in children's blood sugar levels, but they're not quite as bad as table sugar. They also have two added advantages: they do contain some vitamins and minerals, and their stronger taste means you don't have to use so much of them.

Sugary foods should be discouraged in children's diets, but it's pointless trying to ban them outright – children will only find ways to eat them when they're away from home. But it's not so difficult to move the sweeter treats to mealtimes, and gradually blunt your child's sweet tooth by reducing the amount of sugar that your family eats.

Sugar-reducing tips:

▶▶ Dump the fizzy drinks. Some cans of drink contain as much as 13 teaspoons of sugar.

▶▶ Encourage children to drink water, milk or fresh fruit juice diluted with water.

▶▶ Avoid sugar-packed breakfast cereals. Add fruit, chopped nuts, seeds or a little grated high-cocoa-solid chocolate to a low-sugar or no added sugar cereal instead.

▶▶ Make your own low-sugar muesli – children love helping to choose which cereals, dried fruits, nuts and seeds to include. As well as using at breakfast time, it's great sprinkled on desserts – you'll find our muesli recipe suggestion on page 155.

▶▶ Hunt out the low-sugar options when shopping for baked beans, tinned spaghetti, sauces and salad dressings.

▶▶ Offer non-sugar or low-sugar toppings for toast, crackers and sandwiches. Try reduced-sugar peanut butter and jams, cream cheese, hummus or a scraping of yeast extract spread (but go easy on this as it's high in salt).

▶▶ Make a platter of juicy fruit chunks with a couple of tablespoons of natural yogurt or fromage frais your usual dessert after dinner. It's the perfect opportunity to introduce new fruits. Try melon, watermelon, kiwi, apricots, mango, plums, berry fruits, ripe pears and crunchy apple crescents. You can always sweeten the yogurt with some fruit puree, a tiny bit of honey or a teaspoon of reduced-sugar jam.

▶▶ Mash a banana or some fresh berry fruits into a natural yogurt or fromage frais instead of buying ready-made desserts.

▶▶ Develop your child's taste for good-quality chocolate (rather than the ultra-sweet fatty kind) by choosing chocolate with a cocoa-solid content of over 60%. As it is higher in caffeine, avoid giving it in the evening.

▶▶ Keep the lid on the sweetie tin. Only have a few sweets in the house at any time so that children learn that when they're eaten they are gone until the next sweetie-tin top-up.

▶▶ Rather than using shop-bought syrupy ice-cream toppings, whizz mango, berries or other soft fresh fruit, sweetened with a little honey to a puree to make a sauce to pour over set yogurt.

▶▶ Keep a jar of sultanas, raisins, chopped dried ready-to-eat apricots and unsalted nuts in the kitchen. A tablespoon makes a quick snack in place of sweets, at least some of the time.

Good sugars: Sugars occur naturally, as well as being added to foods. When people talk about 'sugar', they generally mean sucrose, or table sugar – the kind that's added to cooking, and to many processed foods. And this is the kind we should try to minimise in our children's diets. But there are other kinds of sugars.

Fruits contain a natural sugar called fructose, while milk contains lactose, or milk sugar. These natural sugars are slowly absorbed by the body, providing a steady, slow release of energy, which is what children need.

Foods containing natural sugars are also healthy in their own right – fruits are packed with loads of other nutrients, such as immune-boosting antioxidants and fibre. Milk is a great source of protein and calcium, and both are packed with vitamins and minerals – a far cry from sugary chocolate bars and fizzy drinks, which have virtually no nutritional benefits at all, in fact quite the opposite!

Looking after children's teeth: Children's second set of teeth are also called their 'permanent' teeth – and this is what they should be. But a recent government survey of dental health in children revealed that 50% of school-aged children suffer from tooth decay, and all too often dentists have to extract children's and teenagers' teeth because they're painful and rotten.

Sugars are the main dietary factor in tooth decay. Each time your child eats sugar, bacteria in plaque (the sticky coating on teeth) feed on the sugar and produce acid, which eats away at their teeth.

When it comes to tooth decay, more important than the amount of sugar that children eat is the frequency. By approximately half an hour after a sugary snack, the acid levels in the mouth have returned to normal, but, each time

sugar is eaten, the plaque bacteria get another meal and your child's teeth get another acid bath!

The worst possible time for children to eat sugar is just before bed, after they've cleaned their teeth. The flow of saliva in the mouth slows down when they're asleep, so it takes longer for the sugars and acid to be rinsed away, and the teeth are under attack for longer.

Added sugars (rather than fruit sugars or milk sugars) are the most damaging. Milk, because it's rich in calcium and vitamin D (both important for healthy bones and teeth), is very tooth-friendly indeed.

Drinks can be particularly dangerous for teeth. Sugar-sweetened squash and fizzy drinks feed the plaque bacteria, and all fizzy drinks (including low-calorie, sugar-free or diet versions) are acidic, so they contribute to tooth erosion in their own right. In fact, any acidic food or drink that comes into contact with your child's teeth can damage them.

The only drinks recommended by dentists for between meals are milk and water. But if you find it difficult to persuade your child to drink enough fluids otherwise, well-diluted fruit juice or squash is less acidic (and so less damaging) than pure juice or 'fizz'.

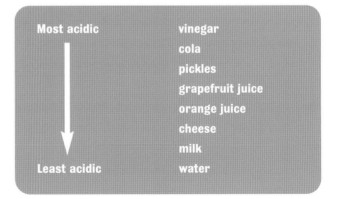

Most acidic	vinegar
	cola
	pickles
	grapefruit juice
	orange juice
	cheese
	milk
Least acidic	water

Top tips for healthy teeth:

▶▶ Keep sweets, and other sugary treats, for eating after meals.

▶▶ Water down pure fruit juice, to make it less acidic and lower the sugar concentration.

▶▶ Offer milk or water as between-meals drinks.

▶▶ When your children do have acidic drinks, such as fruit juice or the occasional glass of fizz or squash, give them a straw to drink through – this keeps the acid away from their teeth.

▶▶ For the same reason, discourage them from swishing acidic drinks around their mouths.

And some non-foodie tips:

▶▶ Children should brush their teeth twice daily with a small blob of fluoride toothpaste.

▶▶ Help your child to make friends with their dentist – six-monthly checkups are recommended.

CHEESE – THE DENTAL DREAM FOOD

Hard cheeses, such as Cheddar, seem to protect children's teeth against tooth decay. Hard cheese is high in fat and salt, so this isn't an excuse for children to guzzle huge quantities of it, but the science suggests that giving your child a small piece of cheese after a meal, or using cheese as a between-meals snack (to replace a sugary snack) could be a good way to help protect their teeth.

Fats

Just like calories and sugars, fats aren't bad in themselves. Yes, fats can cause children to put on weight if they eat too much. But they need a certain amount of fat in their diets:

▶▶ To be broken down to provide fuel for their bodies

▶▶ To keep them warm

▶▶ To absorb and use certain vitamins, such as vitamins A, D, E and K

▶▶ To keep their skin smooth and hair glossy

▶▶ To make hormones

▶▶ For healthy brain development and function – the brain is 60% fat!

Because certain fats are involved in development, it's particularly important for children to get an adequate supply of these ones.

There are good fats and bad fats. While some kinds of fats are bad for our children's health, increasing their risk of diseases such as heart disease in the future, others are positively good for them. We just have to make sure that we minimise our children's intake of the 'unhealthy' kinds of fats, while ensuring that they get enough of the 'healthy' fats.

These are the two main kinds of fats:

▶▶ Saturated fats – 'unhealthy'

▶▶ Unsaturated fats – 'healthy'

Saturated fats

These are mainly animal fats, and are solid at room temperature. Examples include the fat in meat, chicken, cheese and butter. Milk and yoghurt also contain saturated fat, but it's contained in little globules.

Children don't need saturated fats. Everyone can get all the fats they need from unsaturated sources, which are much healthier.

Saturated fats raise the levels of the harmful kind of cholesterol in the blood, which can contribute to clogged arteries. Cholesterol deposits build up gradually over time, and the earlier your arteries start to become clogged with cholesterol deposits, the greater your risk of heart disease or stroke in years to come.

Your child doesn't need to totally avoid saturated fats — after all, they're found in plenty of good, healthy foods, like lean meat, eggs and dairy products. You just have to watch that not too much of their fat intake is coming from these sources, with more coming from the healthy fats that reduce their risk of heart problems later.

Trans fats

If eating too much saturated fat is bad for children, trans fats are even worse. These chemically altered fats find their way into a huge proportion of processed foods, because they're cheap, and keep for ages. They're often used for frying in fast-food outlets. You'll also find them in ready meals, sauces in packets and jars, 'instant' mixes such as soups, drinks and desserts, bought cakes and cake mixes, biscuits, pastries, sweets, desserts, some ice creams, chocolates and chocolate bars.

The best way to minimise the trans fats in your child's diet is to keep it simple, and to make as much as possible from scratch.

Unsaturated fats

All fats – including unsaturated fats – are high in calories, so can cause children to gain weight if they eat too much of them. But unsaturated fats help protect children's health, and they need a certain amount of them in their diets.

Unsaturated fats are generally liquid at room temperature. They include most vegetable oils, and fish oils.

There are two main kinds of unsaturated fats:

▶▶ Poly-unsaturated fats
▶▶ Mono-unsaturated fats

Poly-unsaturated fats:

For example:

▶▶ sunflower oil
▶▶ safflower oil
▶▶ corn oil

Poly-unsaturates are good for children's hearts. They're also involved in growth and development, and can help maintain calm and stable moods. So they're definitely important in any child's diet.

Omega-3 and Omega-6 fatty acids are also poly-unsaturates, and you'll find these in oily fish, nuts and seeds, and green leafy vegetables.

LOOK AT THE LABEL!

You won't see 'trans fats' on the labels – look for the word 'hydrogenated' or 'partially hydrogenated' vegetable fats or oils instead. This means that a food will have trans fats in it.

Mono-unsaturated fats:

For example:

▶▶ olive oil

▶▶ canola oil

▶▶ rapeseed oil

▶▶ peanut oil

Avocados and olives are also high in mono-unsaturated fats, which are also called 'mono-unsaturates'. Mono-unsaturates are even more heart-healthy than poly-unsaturates.

Essential fatty acids: The essential fatty acids, or EFAs, are a special group of poly-unsaturated fats, and there are two main kinds:

▶▶ Omega-3 EFAs

▶▶ Omega-6 EFAs

Omega-3 EFAs: These beneficial fats are good for children's cholesterol levels and blood pressure, which reduce their risk of heart disease and stroke in the future.

The best sources of Omega-3s are oily fish, such as salmon, mackerel, sardines and herring. Fresh oily fish is best, but canned oily fish is a reasonable source, except for tuna, as the Omega-3s are destroyed in the tuna-canning process.

Some non-fish foods also contain Omega-3s, but these are less easy for the body to use. The best vegetarian Omega-3 sources are flax seeds (linseeds) and their oil, but they're also found in pumpkin seeds and walnuts (and their oil), and green leafy vegetables such as kale and spinach.

Nutritionists recommend four servings of fish a week for children. At least one of these should be oily fish, but girls under 16 should have a maximum of two oily fish portions, and boys should have a maximum of four. This is because some oily fish can contain chemicals that could harm children if they eat them in large amounts. We're advised not to give children marlin, swordfish and shark at all, as the concentration of chemicals in their flesh can be particularly high.

Omega-6 EFAs: These healthy fats have similar health effects to Omega-3s, and are particularly good for children's skin, helping to keep it supple and prevent dryness. Omega-6s are found in nuts and seeds, as well as some vegetable oils – corn oil, sunflower oil and safflower oil.

SLIPPERY TIPS

● Store oils in a cool, dark cupboard. Sunlight and warmth can turn them rancid.

● Some oils, such as walnut, flaxseed, pumpkin and avocado oil, aren't suitable for cooking, as heating breaks down their chemical structure, destroying their health benefits. Use them instead to make tasty salad dressings.

● Oils that can stand high temperatures, and are suitable for cooking, include peanut, sunflower, sesame, rapeseed and rice bran oil. Olive can also be used for frying, so long as you're careful not to overheat it. It's particularly suitable for quick stir-fries.

● Buy cold-pressed oil if you can – many of the health-giving properties are lost when heat is used to extract the oil.

● Sesame oil has a particularly nutty taste. It's commonly used in Chinese cookery, and is wonderful in dressings for noodle salads.

Getting the balance right: Most children find it easier to get enough of the Omega-6 EFAs, since they're found in commonly eaten foods like chicken, eggs, sunflower oil and fat spreads. It's harder for them to get enough Omega-3s, as they're found in oily fish, flax seeds and their oil, which don't feature highly in most children's favourites!

Don't get stressed about getting the balance precisely right, though. If you up the Omega-3s in your child's diet, this should help even the balance and take you close to the target.

If your child doesn't like oily fish, you can also boost their intake with special Omega-3-enriched foods such as eggs or milk, or a good-quality Omega-3 or fish-oil supplement (make sure you buy fish oil, *not* fish liver oil or cod liver oil – this is very different).

Getting the amount of fat in a child's diet right is a matter of balance. They need enough to fuel their active little bodies, to keep them warm and to ensure they get enough of the EFAs and the vitamins contained in fats, for healthy growth and development. But, because it's high in calories, too much fat can lead them to put on weight.

Try to ensure that most of the fats in your child's diet are unsaturated fats. Keep an eye on your family's intake of saturated fats, from animal products such as meat and dairy products, by choosing lean cuts of meat and low-fat versions of dairy products.

Trimming unnecessary fat

▶▶ Change to low-fat alternatives of dairy products such as milk, yoghurt and cheese.

▶▶ If you use a strong, tasty cheese, such as mature Cheddar, you won't have to use so much of it.

▶▶ Switch from margarine or butter to low-fat spread – look for one that's low in saturates and high in mono-unsaturates and poly-unsaturates.

▶▶ Serve naturally low-fat foods – fruit, vegetables and grains.

▶▶ Spread sandwiches and rolls with a little low-fat soft cheese or low-fat salad cream – you won't need butter or spread.

▶▶ Serve homemade oven chips and potato wedges instead of chips – you'll find the recipes in Part 5.

▶▶ Pour natural yoghurt or fromage frais over desserts instead of cream.

▶▶ Quark is a low-fat soft cheese which makes a good substitute for whipped or clotted cream on desserts or scones. It tastes mild and extremely creamy.

▶▶ Choose low-fat cooking methods like stir-frying, steaming, poaching and grilling instead of roasting with fat or frying.

▶▶ Trim all visible fat from meat and remove the skin from chicken before cooking – chicken skin is where most of the fat lurks.

▶▶ Grill meat on a rack, or cook on a ridged griddle, so that fat can drain away.

▶▶ Lightly brush meat with oil before cooking rather than putting oil in the pan – you'll use less.

▶▶ Reduce the amount of meat you need in a stew or casserole by adding some tinned beans or lentils.

▶▶ Measure oil into a pan with a spoon rather than adding it straight from the bottle – it's easy to overestimate the amount you need if you do it by eye.

▶▶ Make fast foods an occasional treat, and then choose the healthiest options you can.

▶▶ Give shop-bought and restaurant-bought pizzas with meat and sausage fillings a miss. Choose vegetable and lean chicken or fish toppings, and scrape off some of the cheese if you can. Alternatively make or buy a pizza base and construct your own. Let the children help.

▶▶ Limit high-fat snacks such as chocolate bars, crisps, cakes and biscuits and offer instead currant buns spread with a little low-sugar jam, rice cakes, oatcakes spread with a healthy peanut butter, or fresh fruit.

Fantastic Fibre

Fibre doesn't have a very glamorous image. But there's more to fibre than bran and bowels!

Fibre is important for keeping the digestive system working smoothly, and reduces the risk of certain cancers, such as bowel cancer, later in life.

Fibre also helps fill children up, so they're less likely to want unhealthy snacks between meals.

How much fibre?

There's no official recommended intake of fibre for children, but adults are recommended to eat a minimum of 18g, and children are advised to eat proportionally less, according to their size.

Most children don't eat enough fibre, largely because they rely so much on processed foods, which are generally low in fibre.

Fibre is wonderful stuff and, in order to stay healthy, children need a certain amount of it. But problems can arise if you overdo things. Children who eat a diet that's excessively high in fibre may become full too quickly, so they don't finish their meals, and so miss out on vital nutrients. Fibre also reduces the amount of certain minerals (especially iron) that children absorb from food.

If you're feeding a diet with large amounts of wholegrain foods and pulses, and your child complains of feeling full up before they finish their meals (and you don't suspect they merely want to go and play, or move on to dessert!), the fibre may be filling them too fast. Swap some of the 'brown' products for 'white' products such as 'ordinary' pasta, white bread or white rice, and see if this helps.

Water

Our bodies consist of approximately 65% water, and losing just 1–2% of this can leave children feeling below par, leading to a variety of symptoms, including lack of concentration and 'fuzzy-headedness', 'grouchiness' and headaches.

It's easy for children to get dehydrated. They're less sensitive to thirst than adults – and also more easily distracted by things that seem much more fun than keeping hydrated! You need to keep on encouraging them to drink water (not fizzy drinks or squash!).

Adults are advised to drink approximately 1.5–2 litres of water a day, which amounts to about 8–10 glasses. Children should drink approximately 8–10 small glasses. In hot weather, dry air-conditioned interiors (such as classrooms, shopping centres and aeroplanes), after exercise, or if they've been suffering from diarrhoea or sickness, children need to drink more.

Salt

Most children eat far too much salt – the average child's salt intake is at least twice as high as it should be.

And why is that a bad thing? Because too much salt can

raise blood pressure and increase the risk of heart attacks in the future, they could be storing up health problems for later. Also, salt gives children a taste for salty food, so they're more likely to carry on eating too much salt when they grow up.

Adults are advised to eat no more than 6g of salt per day, but, because children are smaller than we are, they should have less.

> ## RECOMMENDED MAXIMUM INTAKES OF SALT – LESS IS BETTER
>
> 1–3 years – 2g salt a day (0.8g sodium)
> 4–6 years – 3g salt a day (1.2g sodium)
> 7–10 years – 5g salt a day (2g sodium)
> 11+ years – 6g salt a day (2.5g sodium)

And it's not just the salt they sprinkle on their meals that you need to watch out for – an amazing 75% of the salt we eat is 'hidden' in processed foods – so it's important to keep a close eye on the amounts we may be feeding our children. Crisps, savoury snacks and packet and tinned soups are some of the worst culprits but high levels of salt can also be found in foods that are sweet, such as biscuits, cakes and breakfast cereals.

High salt foods – limit these:
- Bacon, soy sauce, cheese, crisps, pretzels, gravy granules, pickles, salted nuts

'Watch out' foods – check the labels, as some brands are much higher in salt than others:

- Baked beans, tinned spaghetti, tomato ketchup, pizzas, ready meals, soups, tinned vegetables, tinned beans and lentils, hot chocolate, breakfast cereals

Of course, it's far better to make your own meals from scratch, rather than relying on bought ready meals, pizzas and soups – then you control the salt. You can also cut the salt in your children's diets by:
- Making homemade cakes and biscuits rather than having bought ones – children love to help.
- Choosing low-salt options for baked beans and tinned spaghetti.

> ## SALT MATHS
>
> It's the sodium in salt that's harmful, and sodium is what many manufacturers print on their labels, so make sure that you know whether you're looking at the salt content, or the sodium content.
>
> You can calculate the salt content of a food by multiplying the sodium by 2.5.
>
> So a food containing 0.5g sodium would contain 1.25g salt.
>
> **This is A LOT of salt**
> 1.25g salt or more per 100g
> (0.5g sodium or more per 100g)
>
> **This is A LITTLE salt**
> 0.25g salt or less per 100g
> (0.1g sodium or less per 100g)

▶▶ Having takeaway meals, which are often high in salt, only very occasionally.

▶▶ Gradually reducing the amount of salt you add during cooking.

▶▶ Experimenting with herbs, spices and reduced-salt soy sauce to add flavour to your cooking, instead of using salt.

▶▶ Not adding salt at the table. Or at least tasting the food first – it probably won't need it.

Vitamins and Minerals

Vitamins and minerals are called 'micronutrients', because we only need them in tiny amounts. But they're huge in terms of importance.

They're needed to make enzymes, which act as catalysts, like tiny spark plugs setting off vital chemical reactions in our bodies. They're also involved in making hormones, which direct a whole range of body processes.

And some minerals, such as iron, calcium and phosphorus, are incorporated into the structure of our bodies, in blood cells, bones and teeth.

Some nutrients are particularly important for children.

STAR NUTRIENTS FOR CHILDREN

- **Omega-3 EFAs for brain function**
- **Calcium for bones and teeth**
- **Iron for energy and muscles**
- **Zinc for a strong immune system**
- **Vitamin C to defend against infection and help wound healing**

Iron

Growing children need iron in order to build muscle, and also to make the red blood cells that ferry oxygen around the body. A deficiency in iron can lead to anaemia, which causes symptoms of tiredness, weakness and poor concentration. A child suffering from anaemia almost certainly won't be doing themselves justice at school.

Iron is found in both animal and vegetarian foods (see table page 30), but it's easier for the body to absorb and use the iron from animal sources. You can increase the amount of iron that children absorb from their food by giving them foods rich in vitamin C at the same time – a small glass of vitamin C-rich orange juice with a meal will do the trick. However, other compounds in foods, such as the tannin in tea, hinder the uptake of iron, and for this reason it's best for children not to have tea at mealtimes.

Calcium

Calcium is needed for healthy bones and teeth. It's important for children to build up their bones as much as possible because, by the time they hit their twenties, they reach their peak bone density, and, from their thirties, bone density slowly but surely decreases. As the bones gradually become thinner, the disease osteoporosis becomes a risk in old age, particularly for women. But building up as much strong healthy bone as possible during childhood leads to the maximum possible 'bone bank', and reduces the risk of osteoporosis later on.

Calcium from dairy products, such as milk, yoghurt and cheese, is easiest for the body to absorb and use. But children can also get this mineral from canned fish where the soft bones are eaten (such as salmon and sardines), and to a lesser extent from sesame seeds, other nuts and seeds, and green leafy vegetables.

Zinc

Zinc is crucial for growth and development, and also helps maintain a healthy immune system, protecting children from all those bugs and germs doing the rounds at school.

The best sources are seeds, nuts and wholegrains, though zinc is also found in green leafy vegetables and pulses.

So, what vitamins and minerals do children need, and where can you find them?

Vitamin	What does it do?	Animal sources	Non-animal sources
Vitamin A	Healthy vision and skin, and a strong immune system	Liver, oily fish, dairy products and eggs	Green vegetables (eg spinach, broccoli), yellow and orange fruit and vegetables (eg cantaloupe melon, apricots, peaches, carrots, sweet potatoes)
B Vitamins (Vitamins B1, B2, B3, B6, B12)	Releasing energy from food. Making blood cells. Keeping the nervous system healthy	Meat, fish, dairy products, eggs	Wholegrains, pulses (beans and lentils), nuts, seeds, yeast extract, vegetables
Folic acid (another B vitamin)	Helps the body to absorb nutrients effectively, and supports the immune system.	Liver, eggs	Green leafy vegetables, fortified breakfast cereals, pulses (beans and lentils), nuts, citrus fruit, broccoli, brown rice, wheatgerm
Vitamin C	Keeps the immune system strong, and is needed for healing. Helps the body to absorb iron from food		Fruit (especially kiwifruit, blackcurrants, strawberries, citrus fruits), yellow and red peppers, tomatoes, Brussels sprouts
Vitamin D	Vital for healthy bones and teeth, as it helps the body absorb and use calcium	Oily fish (eg salmon, sardines, mackerel), meat, eggs, dairy products	A chemical reaction caused by the action of sunlight on the skin enables the body to make vitamin D
Vitamin E	Supports the immune system, protects the body's cells		Nuts and seeds and their oils, wholemeal bread, wheatgerm, avocado, spinach, broccoli
Vitamin K	Helping blood to clot, and for healthy bones	Eggs, fish oils, dairy products	Green leafy vegetables

Mineral	Role	Animal sources	Non-animal sources
Iron	Production of healthy red blood cells and prevention of anaemia	Liver (the best source), kidney, red meat	Pulses (beans and lentils), green vegetables, dried fruit (especially apricots)
Calcium	Building and maintaining healthy bones and teeth. Helps muscles to function properly	Dairy foods, tinned fish where the bones are eaten (eg sardines & salmon)	Tofu, sesame seeds, almonds, figs, kale and other green leafy vegetables
Zinc	Supporting the immune system and preventing infection, healthy growth and development	Oysters, meat, fish, chicken, eggs, dairy products	Seeds (especially pumpkin seeds), nuts, wholegrains, green leafy vegetables, beans and lentils
Magnesium	Helps the body deal with stress and for muscle function. Also needed for healthy bones		Green vegetables, nuts and seeds, pulses, wholegrains, dried fruits

Supplements

In theory, children shouldn't need supplements – they should get all the vitamins and minerals they need from their healthy food. Also, the vitamins and minerals in real food are better absorbed and easier for the body to use.

But that's not to say that supplements don't have a place. In practice, it can be extremely difficult to reach all of the recommended daily amounts, even if you strive to give your child a balanced diet.

There's nothing wrong with giving your child a quality brand of multivitamin supplement that's specially designed for children, to top up any micronutrient 'gaps' in your child's diet. But supplements should always be a last resort, rather than a first choice. A pill is no substitute for a healthy diet of fresh food, but it can give you peace of mind if, for example, your child doesn't manage to hit their 'five-a-day' target every day.

Remember, though, that vitamins and minerals are powerful things, and some of them can build up to potentially harmful levels in a child's body if taken in excess. For this reason, make sure that any supplement you give your child contains no more than 100% of the recommended daily amount (RDA) for the vitamins and minerals. You should also avoid giving 'single' vitamins or minerals (such as a supplement of vitamin C or the B vitamins, or iron) as well as a multivitamin, except under medical advice.

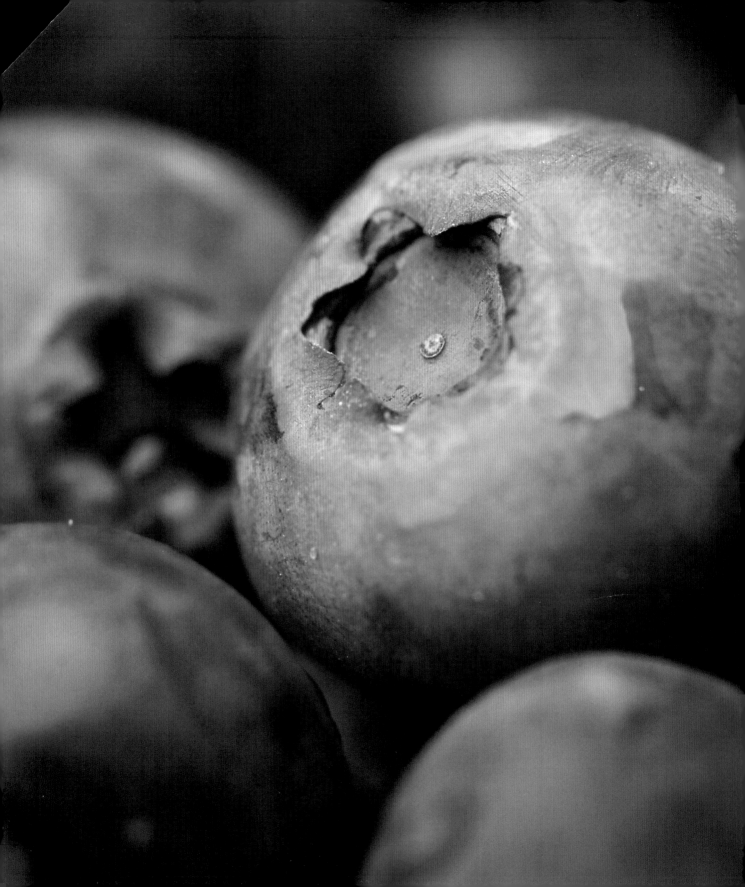

CHAPTER THREE

FOODS FOR CHILDREN

A healthy diet for children (and everyone) can be summed up in two words – balance and variety.

Balance: Plenty of the really healthy foods, with only a little of the less healthy ones.

Variety: Different foods contain different nutrients, so giving your child a really varied diet maximises their chances of getting all the nutrients they need.

fabulous fruit and vital vegetables

Fruit and vegetables are true superfoods. They contain:

▶▶ Vitamins – they're particularly good for vitamin C and folic acid

▶▶ Minerals – many are a great source of potassium

▶▶ Phytochemicals (plant chemicals), such as the antioxidants that defend our bodies from damage

▶▶ Soluble fibre, for heart health

▶▶ Insoluble fibre, for digestive health

▶▶ Natural sugars, for energy

▶▶ Water, to help top up hydration levels

They're low in fat and salt (unless you add it to them when cooking), so they're good for children to snack on without putting on weight.

Getting your 'five-a-day'

All of us – children included – are encouraged to eat at least five portions of fruit and vegetables a day. But fewer than one in five children reach their five-a-day target. What counts towards five-a-day?

▶▶ Fresh fruit and vegetables

▶▶ Frozen fruit and vegetables

FIVE A DAY QUIZ

Take our quiz to see how your child is doing. Just fill in the number of portions they ate yesterday.

FRUIT

☐ How many portions of fresh fruit?

☐ How many portions of tinned fruit?

☐ How many portions of canned fruit?

☐ How many portions of dried fruit (maximum of one)?

☐ How many glasses of fruit juice (maximum of one)?

☐ TOTAL

VEGETABLES

☐ How many portions of fresh vegetables?

☐ How many portions of tinned vegetables?

☐ How many portions of frozen vegetables?

☐ How many portions of baked beans in tomato sauce (maximum of one)?

☐ TOTAL

☐ GRAND TOTAL OF FRUIT + VEGETABLES

Most children score higher for fruit than vegetables, but you should really aim for a minimum of two portions of fruit, and at least three vegetable portions. This is because, as a rule, vegetables are slightly more nutritious, and it's harder to get children to eat them, so we have to make more effort!

▶▶ Canned fruit and vegetables

▶▶ One portion of dried fruit such as raisins, sultanas, dried apricots or dried apples (any further portions don't count)

▶▶ Beans such as kidney beans

▶▶ One small (150ml) glass of fruit juice (any further fruit juice drunk doesn't count)

▶▶ One portion of baked beans in tomato sauce (it's the tomato that makes it count)

Even though they're officially vegetables, potatoes don't add to your five-a-day total – they're counted as a starchy carbohydrate food.

fabulous fruit
What counts as a child-sized portion?

As a rough guide, a portion is the amount of fruit that will fit into a child's hand – so the portion size grows with the child.

But just as a guideline, here are a few ideas for child-sized portions to count towards that five-a-day:

▶▶ A small apple, banana or peach

▶▶ 10–12 grapes

▶▶ 1 Mandarin or Clementine

▶▶ 1 kiwifruit, dessert plum or Satsuma

▶▶ A slice of melon or pineapple

▶▶ 7 strawberries

▶▶ 2–3 tablespoons of drained tinned fruit

▶▶ A small glass of pure fruit juice (diluted with water)

▶▶ 1 tablespoon of raisins or sultanas

▶▶ 3 ready-to-eat dried apricots, sliced

FRESH, FROZEN OR CANNED?

In an ideal world, we'd all feed our families fresh fruit and vegetables straight from the ground or tree.

But life's not like that. Few of us can grow more than a small proportion of the fruit and veg we eat, and the produce you see in the supermarket could have been harvested several weeks ago, and its vitamin content will have deteriorated over time.

But, when you freeze or can foods, the nutrient loss is stopped in its tracks.

Frozen foods are flash-frozen soon after harvesting, minimising vitamin loss. Fruits and vegetables are boiled during canning, so much of their B vitamins and vitamin C dissolves into the canning liquid. Often, this is highly sugared or salted, which means that, if you use the liquid (and the vitamins), you get the sugar or salt as well.

Eat a rainbow

It's best for children to eat as many *different* fruit and vegetables as possible. Different fruit and veg contain different combinations of vitamins, minerals and phytochemicals (plant chemicals), so this gives children a wider variety of nutrients.

A great way to help children to eat a variety of fruit and vegetables is to encourage them to 'eat a rainbow'. Children love charts, so, as a way of getting them to eat fruit and vegetables, design a chart and let them fill in the different colour vegetables they eat each day. Here are just a few ideas:

Red: Cherries, strawberries, plums, tomatoes, red peppers, radishes

Orange: Oranges, apricots, mangoes, melon, sweet potatoes

Yellow: Yellow peppers, pineapples, butternut squash, sweetcorn

Green: Broccoli, peas, courgettes, green grapes, kiwifruit

Blue: Blueberries, black grapes, plums

Indigo (or black): Aubergines, blackberries, blackcurrants

Violet (or purple): Red cabbage, beetroot

Not forgetting white: Cauliflower, onions, leeks, turnips, mushrooms

Eating more fruit

Getting children to eat fruit is generally easier than persuading them to eat vegetables. It's sweeter, juicier, brightly coloured and often simpler to eat raw. But today's children think that fresh fruit is 'sour', because they're used to processed foods with loads of sugar and artificial sweeteners added. There's a simple way to help prevent their taste buds becoming 'sugar saturated' – cut back on the sugary and artificially sweetened foods, particularly sweets.

Ways to get children to eat more fruit
Serving ideas

▸▸ Make sure that the fruit you serve is ripe or it will be hard and tasteless, and may cause tummy upsets – a sure way for a child to decide they don't like that particular fruit.

▸▸ To stop fruits such as apples and pears turning brown (which could put children off), and also to preserve their vitamin C, cut them just before you are ready to use them.

▶▶ If you're going on a journey, pack a lidded plastic container with apple slices, grapes and orange segments for a healthy snack in the car. Don't forget to pack some wet wipes for sticky fingers.

▶▶ Wedges of watermelon make a great addition to a picnic and most children love the sweet, juicy taste (and spitting out the seeds!).

▶▶ Offer thin slices of cheese and pear or apple slices at the end of a meal.

▶▶ Add fresh or dried fruit to breakfast cereals.

▶▶ Cut kiwifruits in half, put them in an eggcup, and let the children eat them like a boiled egg, with a spoon.

Shopping ideas

▶▶ Buy fruit a little at a time, if you can, to avoid waste. Or buy it under-ripe and ripen it at home.

▶▶ Ring the changes by serving fruits as they come into season, along with exotic fruits when there isn't much British fruit.

▶▶ When you're shopping with the children, let each of them choose one piece of fruit to take home for a snack.

Snack ideas

▶▶ Prepare a platter of fruit for them to dip into when they come home from school. They're often really hungry at this time, so it's a good time to slip in an unfamiliar fruit.

▶▶ Don't give up if the first time you introduce a new fruit they decide they don't like it. Offer it again a few weeks later, perhaps cutting it in a different way.

▶▶ Have a fruit bowl in the house to encourage children to snack on fruit instead of biscuits or sweets.

Dessert ideas

Most children love desserts, so it's a great opportunity to get fruit inside them.

▶▶ If you're serving a fruit dessert after dinner, put some slices of a new fruit on a separate plate and tell them you bought it just for yourself. A sure-fire way to make them ask to try it because they think they might be missing something!

▶▶ Make fruit special – serve it layered in glasses with yogurt or fromage frais. If your child finds natural yogurt too sour, sweeten it with some honey or a little bit of grated good-quality chocolate.

▶▶ Purée fruit, with a little sugar if necessary. Put a scoop of low-fat Quark (a soft cheese), some fromage frais or yoghurt on a plate and pour the purée around to form a moat.

▶▶ Warmed fruit purée poured over a homemade mini muffin makes a special dessert.

▶▶ Slice pineapple and banana, sprinkle over a little brown sugar or caster sugar, and grill or bake until the sugar melts. Keep your eye on it as the sugar burns easily and it could become bitter. Serve with a spoonful of low-fat fromage frais.

▶▶ Fill homemade or bought pancakes with fruit or fruit purée.

▶▶ Serve grilled or baked fruit with Scotch pancakes and low-fat fromage frais.

▶▶ For older children, make kebabs from chunks of fruit threaded on to skewers and lightly grill them. Pineapple, pear, nectarine, mango and peach work really well.

▶▶ Make fresh fruit juice and smoothies to introduce new fruit tastes.

▶▶ Low-fat rice pudding with a couple of spoonfuls of stewed fruit or purée makes a healthy dessert and children love stirring the fruit through the rice pudding to see it change colour. Try stewed plums or puréed tinned apricots.

▶▶ Make fruit crumbles with an oaty topping.

▶▶ Add fresh fruit to jellies.

Growing ideas

▶▶ Let the children grow strawberries. All you need are a few plant pots.

▶▶ If you have a garden, grow a few fruit bushes, raspberry or blackberry canes. Children love watching the fruit develop and picking it when it's ripe.

A NOTE ON DRIED FRUIT

When you're buying dried fruit, it's a good idea to pay a little bit extra for quality, if you can. Dried fruit is often treated with chemicals, such as the preservative sulphur dioxide which is used to extend its shelf life, and make the fruit look more attractive. For example, 'treated' dried apricots look orange and, well, more 'apricoty', while organic, unsulphured apricots are dark brown, and don't look much like apricots at all. But they taste just as good, or better.

Try to buy organic dried fruit whenever possible, because sulphur dioxide isn't allowed in organic fruit.

▶▶ Make use of 'Pick your Own' growers and farmers' markets. Children will love picking fruit straight from the plants into a basket. Just try to make sure that more ends up inside the baskets than in the children, to prevent upset stomachs later on!

▶▶ For more tips on getting children interested in growing food, turn to Part 3.

vital veggies

Most children like fruit, but persuading them to eat vegetables may prove trickier. This is a pity, because many of the compounds that make vegetables less sweet and more bitter than fruit are super-nutrients with impressive properties, such as helping to prevent chronic diseases like cancer and heart disease later in life. Here's an example – the slightly bitter compound that puts the 'yuk factor' (for some children at least) in broccoli is one of the reasons it's so good for them!

Getting children to eat their vegetables can be a challenge – particularly if the vegetable happens to be green! This is where you may need to employ a wide variety of strategies and even engage in a little stealth. It's surprisingly simple to sneak vegetables into pasta sauces, soups, mashed potato, stews and casseroles.

By the time they reach five or six years old, children may decide it's time to refuse to eat certain foods, particularly if it seems really important to you that they eat them! If an older brother or sister has decided they no longer eat vegetables, younger ones may follow suit. Don't panic or make a big deal of it. But don't give up – staying calm and persevering generally pays off in the end.

Your own example is crucial when persuading children that vegetables are good things to eat. If they see that the adults in the household don't eat them, why should they?

Fortunately there's a wide variety of colourful, tasty fresh, frozen and tinned vegetables on offer today. We can't expect children to like all of them, but we won't know what they do like if they're not offered. You might be in for a pleasant surprise.

Getting children to eat vegetables
Shopping and growing tips
▶▶ Get enthusiastic when you see a new vegetable in the supermarket and suggest buying some to try.
▶▶ Try out 'exotic' vegetables, such as sweet potatoes and mooli (a kind of giant radish).
▶▶ Let the children take turns to choose a new vegetable when you go shopping.
▶▶ Let children grow cress on damp kitchen paper in a see-through plastic container (the kind supermarkets often use for soft fruit, tomatoes and mushrooms are ideal). Children enjoy watching the seeds grow and harvesting the cress with scissors. Use the cress in salads and sandwich fillings.

Serving tips
▶▶ Introduce new vegetables on a regular basis so that children become used to seeing new foods on the table. If they don't like them first time round, persevere. But don't force them to try something new or offer a bribe.
▶▶ Have a bowl of salad on the table at mealtimes so that children can dip into it. A selection of Little Gem lettuce leaves, celery sticks, wedges of tomato and slices of cucumber are popular choices.
▶▶ Keep a bowl of veggie sticks handy in the fridge for nibbles. Also have them on hand when children are watching TV. They might even dip in and eat them without even realising they're eating vegetables.
▶▶ Children love dipping. Serve lightly cooked cauliflower and broccoli florets, carrot sticks, asparagus, celery sticks or French beans with a low-fat dip.
▶▶ The skin is often the least tasty part of a tomato. So if your children say they don't like tomatoes, try removing the skins. If that doesn't work, try removing the skins and the seeds.
▶▶ Sprinkle grated cheese and wholemeal breadcrumbs over vegetables and pop under the grill until it is golden. The crunchy, savoury topping will give the dish a whole new look and taste.

Cooking tips
▶▶ Vary your cooking methods. Try steaming, boiling, stir-frying, baking and grilling vegetables.
▶▶ Let the children get involved. At the weekend make or buy mini pizza bases. Make a fresh tomato sauce, grate some cheese and lay out a selection of veggie toppings, so they can make their own individual pizzas.
▶▶ Or add a few more veggie toppings to shop-bought low-fat and low-salt pizzas. Try some peas, sliced mushrooms, sweetcorn, tomato slices or peppers.
▶▶ Children often like foods that are crisp. Grate par-boiled potatoes and carrots, combine with mashed sweetcorn, and drop tablespoons into a lightly oiled non-stick pan to make little low-fat veggie fritters. Cook until the

fritters are golden brown on both sides. Ring the changes by adding a few peas to the mixture.

▶▶ Make veggie cakes by combining mashed cooked boiled potatoes, carrots, cabbage and sweetcorn.

Don't let your roasting repertoire end with potatoes!

ROASTED ROOTS

Oven-roast chunky sticks or wedges of carrot, swede and parsnip. Simply toss them in a teaspoon of olive oil and bake in a moderate oven until they are tender.

SWEET SESAME PARSNIPS

Parsnips have a naturally sweet taste. Take some small parsnips, remove the hard cores and cut into wedges. Toss in a teaspoon of oil and place on a baking tray. Sprinkle over some sesame seeds and black pepper. Bake in a moderate oven until the parsnips are tender and the sesame seeds are toasted and golden.

MEDITERRANEAN VEGETABLES

Try roast Mediterranean veg – oven-roast chunks of red pepper, wedges of onion (the red ones are sweetest), halved mushrooms and circles of courgette. Toss with a little olive oil, sprinkle with black pepper and bake in a moderate oven until they are tender. These are delicious served hot as a meal accompaniment or used to fill pitta breads, or as a topping for pizzas and on toasted slices of ciabatta or French bread.

Form into little round patties and dust with flour. Cook in a lightly oiled pan until they are golden brown on both sides. Serve with cold cooked chicken and a salad for a quick meal.

▶▶ Serve red cabbage and apple lightly cooked in some low-salt stock. It tastes sweet and won't seem like cabbage to the child.

▶▶ Stuffed tomatoes, small peppers or pieces of hollowed-out courgette filled with sweetcorn and a mixture of breadcrumbs and grated cheese are often popular with children.

▶▶ If your child won't eat boiled Brussels sprouts, try slicing them finely and adding to stir-fries or salads.

Veggies around the world

Have a 'foreign' food meal. For example, choose Chinese, and serve a stir-fry using a combination of Chinese vegetables, such as pak choi or Chinese greens and beansprouts, together with sliced pepper, onions and mushroom. Add some stir-fried slices of chicken or some prawns and serve with rice. Tell the children, 'This is what children eat in China,' let them eat the food out of bowls, and have fun trying to eat with chopsticks.

You could also have an Indian meal of a mild vegetable and chicken curry and rice, or an Italian meal of a pasta dish or a homemade pizza and salad. The variety is endless and the children will think it's fun and different.

Top of the chip parade

Thought chips would be banned in the 6-Week Junk-Free Plan? Not all chips are created equal in the health stakes, and some can be a tasty part of a healthy diet.

Take a look at our league table of chips – number 1 is the healthiest.

But remember that, with shop-bought chips, you need to look carefully at the labelling. Look for those that are low in saturated fat, and that don't contain hydrogenated or partially hydrogenated vegetable oils (which means they'll contain trans fats). If the chips contain saturated or hydrogenated fats, send them a few places down our league table!

1. Homemade Baked Chunky Chips (see Recipes Section in Part 5)
2. Bought oven or microwave chips (thick cut)
3. Bought oven or microwave chips (crinkle cut)
4. Bought oven or microwave chips (thin cut/French fries)
5. Bought chips for frying – you can make sure that you use a mono-unsaturated oil that can take very high temperatures for frying (such as canola or groundnut). Drain the chips well afterwards to remove as much of the fat as possible
6. Bought chips with crispy coating or flavourings – they'll generally contain trans fats and loads of artificial additives
7. Chips from the chip shop – often greasy and fried in hydrogenated vegetable fat
8. Burger-bar French fries – they're thin cut, so soak up more oil, which is often the unhealthy hydrogenated kind

Secret vegetables

Although the ideal is for your child to enjoy vegetables and eat them by choice, it's not the end of the world if they flatly refuse one or more of them. There are plenty of clever ways to slip them into their diet, by mixing them in with foods that are generally popular with children.

▶▶ Add finely chopped, grated or puréed vegetables to pasta sauces, stews or casseroles. Sweet peppers, carrots, courgettes, French beans, cauliflower, broccoli, mushrooms and peas work well.
▶▶ Add a tablespoon of puréed carrots or peas to gravy.
▶▶ Add puréed cauliflower to mashed potato.

marvellous meat and poultry

Meat is a great source of protein in a form that's easy for the body to use. It's also rich in iron, zinc and B vitamins.

But it also contains saturated fat, which we need to minimise in our children's diets.

You can get the goodness of meat, while keeping saturated fat to a minimum, by choosing low-fat meat and cuts.

▶▶ White meats such as chicken or turkey are lower in fat than red meats.
▶▶ Remove the fat from red meat.
▶▶ Remove the skin from poultry.
▶▶ Duck and goose is much fattier than other poultry – go for chicken or turkey.
▶▶ Bought mince often has a lot of fat 'minced in'. Buy inexpensive cuts of lean meat, and mince it yourself.
▶▶ Venison is lower in fat than other red meats.
▶▶ Buy low-fat sausages (look for 5–10% fat) rather than 'ordinary' sausages.

Above all, use 'real' meat rather than processed meat products wherever you can. Processed meat and poultry products are generally high in fat, and many contain a lot of added salt, water, fillers and artificial additives.

> **Where's the fat in chicken?**
> **Grilled chicken breast = 1.7% fat**
> **Chicken skin = 40% fat**

You can also make low-fat versions of your children's fast-food favourites, such as burgers and chicken nuggets – you'll find the recipes in Part 5.

fantastic fish

Fish has a lot going for it – we should encourage our children to eat more! It's high in protein, and rich in the minerals zinc and selenium (for strong immune defences) and iodine (for healthy growth). White fish such as cod, haddock and sole, and prawns, are extremely low in fat. And, while oily fish (salmon, mackerel, sardines and the like) has a higher fat content, it's the healthy poly-unsaturated type that's good for our children's hearts and brains. Oily fish is also a great source of vitamins A and D.

Fish is 'fast food'

Fish is wonderfully quick to cook – the biggest mistake people make is to overcook it, which spoils the flavour and texture.

The healthiest ways to cook fish are:

▶▶ Grilling

> **White fish such as haddock is a great low-fat protein source – it contains a mere 0.6g of fat per 100g, and only 0.1g of that is the harmful saturated kind of fat.**

▶▶ Microwaving
▶▶ Steaming
▶▶ Baking in foil or greaseproof paper parcels
▶▶ Flash-frying – the low-fat way

Flash-frying fish

▶▶ Wipe a frying pan with oil. Seal the fish on a moderate heat and then reduce to a low heat to cook through.
▶▶ When cooked the flesh appears opaque. Fresh salmon turns a pale-pink colour when it is cooked.
▶▶ To test, insert a fork into the thickest part of the flesh and gently divide. It's cooked if it flakes easily. With whole fish, the flesh should fall easily off the backbone.
▶▶ Serve as soon as possible, and remember that fish continues to cook even after it's removed from the heat.

> **Tinned oily fish where the bones are eaten, such as sardines and salmon, also contain calcium.**

good eggs

Eggs are a great food for children.

▶▶ They're a good source of easily absorbed protein.
▶▶ They're lower in fat than meat and chicken, and most of that fat is the heart-healthy mono-unsaturated kind.
▶▶ They won't bust the calorie bank – a medium egg contains 76 calories, about the same as a banana.
▶▶ They're rich in vitamins A, D and E and the B vitamins.
▶▶ They're a good source of minerals, including phosphorus for healthy bones and teeth, and iodine for making the thyroid hormone.

▶▶ They also contain the immune-boosting minerals zinc and selenium.

glorious grains

Slow-release starchy carbohydrates, and especially wholegrains, are great fuel for children. Wholegrains contain all of the goodness of the grain – the protein- and nutrient-rich 'germ' which would grow into a new plant; the fibre-rich bran outer layer; and the starchy layer that would provide energy for the growing seed. When grains are refined to make products such as white flour, the germ and the bran are removed – along with their nutrients and fibre content.

Wholegrains are great sources of:

▶▶ B vitamins (including folic acid)
▶▶ Vitamin E
▶▶ Iron
▶▶ Zinc
▶▶ Magnesium
▶▶ Selenium

You can boost your child's wholegrain intake by giving them wholemeal bread (not 'brown' bread, as this can just be white bread with colouring added!), brown pasta and brown rice.

pulse power

Pulses – beans and lentils – are a fantastic low-fat way to give your child protein and are also a rich source of fibre, including the soluble fibre that's so good for heart health, and high in vitamins, minerals and phytochemicals.

WHOLEGRAIN TIPS

● Have wholegrain cereal for breakfast (look for varieties that are also low in sugar and salt).
● Even better, have porridge or no-sugar, no-salt muesli. Add some fresh fruit and yoghurt to liven it up.
● Have wholegrain crackers rather than cream crackers.
● Where practical, use wholemeal flour (or a mixture of wholemeal and white) in baking.
● Add oats to crumble toppings to boost their fibre content and for added crunch.

Lentils

▶▶ Red lentils – very quick to cook.
▶▶ Continental lentils and puy lentils – fairly quick to cook, and you can also buy them in tins.

Beans

▶▶ Red kidney beans – dark red-brown, and hold their shape well, so they're great for bean salads and chilli con carne.
▶▶ Chick peas – round, and cream in colour, with a nutty taste. Used in hot dishes and cold salads, and puréed to make hummus.
▶▶ Black-eyed beans – white beans with a black 'eye' where they were attached to the pod.
▶▶ Pinto beans – a South American bean with a fluffy texture.

SOYA – THE SUPERBEAN!

Soya beans are even richer in protein than other beans, and are also a good source of iron and calcium. They're very time consuming to prepare from 'dried', but fortunately you can buy them in tins (and they're just as nutritious like this).

You can also get the goodness of soya beans from soya-based products such as tofu (soya bean curd) and vegetarian meat substitutes such as soya mince, soya chunks and soya burgers (check the labelling to see that they're not too high in fat and salt). Soya milk is also made from soya beans – but don't worry, you wouldn't know it from the taste!

▶▶ Borlotti beans – Italian beans with a mild flavour.

▶▶ Dried beans take ages to soak and cook – so buy them in tins for convenience.

▶▶ Use beans or lentils to replace some of the meat in traditional casseroles, stews and curries. You'll slash the amount of saturated fat in the recipe, and boost the fibre, mineral and phytochemical content at the same time.

▶▶ Make a tasty dip or sandwich spread by puréeing beans or lentils with a tiny bit of olive oil, perhaps a dash of lemon or lime juice, and seasoning to taste.

What about quorn?

Quorn isn't a pulse – it's made from so-called mycoprotein, which comes from a kind of fungus (a member of the mushroom family).

Strictly speaking, Quorn is a 'processed food', but it can be a very good and convenient low-fat protein source for children. You just need to check the labelling for salt, fat and additives, as the amounts can sometimes be high. Quorn is available in lots of different forms, such as mince, chunks and 'fillets', which you can use in your own recipes instead of meat, as well as ready-meals, 'sausages', 'grills', burgers and even substitutes for sliced meats for sandwiches.

nifty nuts and seeds

Nuts and seeds aren't just tasty – they're also high in many important nutrients, especially the heart-healthy ones.

▶▶ Protein

▶▶ Mono-unsaturated fats

▶▶ Poly-unsaturated fats

▶▶ Omega-3 and Omega-6 fatty acids

▶▶ B vitamins

▶▶ Magnesium

▶▶ Zinc

▶▶ Fibre

Different nuts and seeds contain different nutrients, so give your child a wide variety in order to get the full range.

NO SALT PLEASE!

Rather than buying salted nuts, buy them 'plain' and roast them in the oven (check them frequently to see they don't burn) or toast them in a dry frying plan. It brings out the flavour.

Peanut power

Most children adore peanut butter (although remember that some can be dangerously allergic to it). Peanut butter is a good source of protein, fibre, vitamins and minerals. It's high in fat (generally around 50% fat) and calories (around 92 calories per tablespoon). That said, over 70% of that fat is the healthy unsaturated kind, so let your child enjoy it in moderation.

Crunchy or smooth, it really doesn't matter, but choose a brand with reduced sugar and salt.

Or make your own healthier version – simply put the peanuts in a grinder and process to the desired texture. You must keep homemade peanut butter in the fridge, and use it within a week, as it won't contain any preservatives and can quickly go rancid.

▶▶ Ring the changes – buy or make different nut butters, such as walnut, almond or cashew nut butter.

▶▶ Or try tahini, a paste made from sesame seeds.

Portion control

Nuts and seeds are little powerhouses of nutrition. But they're also a high-fat food – even healthy fats are high in calories. Include them in your child's diet every day if possible, but keep the portions small, for example the amount your child can fit in the palm of their hand, generally about a dessertspoonful (so bigger children have bigger portions than smaller children).

delightful dairy

Dairy products, such as milk, yoghurt, fromage frais and cheese, are a great source of protein, vitamins and minerals, especially B vitamins, vitamin A, calcium and phosphorus. Just remember that a lot of the fat in dairy products is saturated, so it's best to choose semi-skimmed or skimmed milk, and low-fat dairy products.

Three portions of dairy food – for example, 150ml semi-skimmed milk, a 125g pot of yoghurt and a 25g piece of cheese – provides a child with all of his or her calcium requirement for the day. It also gives them more than 60% of their requirement for vitamin B2, nearly 40% of their vitamin B3, nearly 30% of their folic acid and approximately 20% of their vitamin A, vitamin B1 and vitamin B12 needs.

It's really not that difficult to incorporate three dairy portions into your child's day.

Simple ideas

▶▶ Milk on breakfast cereal or in porridge.

▶▶ A yoghurt or fromage frais in a lunchbox, or as a dessert for dinner.

▶▶ A piece of cheese as a snack or in a lunchbox.

▶▶ A glass of milk when they get home from school (most children prefer milk that is well chilled).

Meal ideas

▶▶ Beat a little milk instead of butter into mashed potato for a smooth and creamy taste.

▶▶ Add milk to homemade soups just before serving.

Dessert ideas

▶▶ Cut a banana into slices and pile up into towers in a bowl. Pour over homemade custard.

▶▶ Serve low-fat rice pudding with fresh, frozen or tinned fruit, or fruit purée.

Snack ideas

▶▶ Don't stick to Cheddar – introduce children to new cheeses. Select a day as 'cheese-tasting day'. Buy

---

CHOOSING YOUR CHEESE

Which cheese is best for your child? It's hard to say – they all have their selling points.

Hard cheeses (Cheddar, Danish Blue, Parmesan)

● Higher in vitamins A, D and E than soft cheese but also higher in saturated fat.

● Among the hard cheeses, Edam is one of the lowest in fat.

● Parmesan has a very strong taste – so you only need to add a little bit to give a dish a cheesy flavour, cutting the fat content in the process.

Soft cheeses (Brie, Camembert, Mozzarella, cream cheese)

● Lower in vitamins A, D and E than soft cheese but also lower in saturated fat.

● Full-fat cream cheese is almost as high in fat as most hard cheeses – so go for the low-fat soft cheeses.

● Cheese spread (especially low-fat versions) is lower in fat than cream cheese. But watch out for those with lots of added salt and other additives.

● Children who don't like the taste of other 'cheesier' cheeses may enjoy cottage cheese with its milder taste.

---

small pieces of two or three cheeses they haven't tasted and serve them with small crackers or pieces of oatcake and some chutney as an after-school treat.

▶▶ Add a few sticks of cheese to a pot of crunchy vegetable sticks. Try cucumber, carrots and celery sticks.

▶▶ Cottage cheese with pineapple and oatcakes makes a good after-school snack, too.

Whole, semi- or skimmed – which milk to choose?

Very young children (between the ages of one and two) should have whole (full-fat) milk, as they need the calories and nutrients it contains, but they can be gradually moved on to semi-skimmed as they get older.

Semi-skimmed milk is best for primary-school-aged children, unless your doctor advises you to switch to skimmed for weight-loss reasons. This is because semi-skimmed milk is a richer source of vitamins A, D and E, which are particularly important for children. These vitamins are fat-soluble – they're found in the fatty component of milk, most of which is removed if the milk is skimmed.

Dairy alternatives

If your child can't have dairy products, for example if they're lactose intolerant, there are plenty of alternatives. Look for those that are fortified with vitamins and minerals, especially calcium.

And there's no reason why these delicious drinks can't be enjoyed by everyone, not just children who can't drink milk.

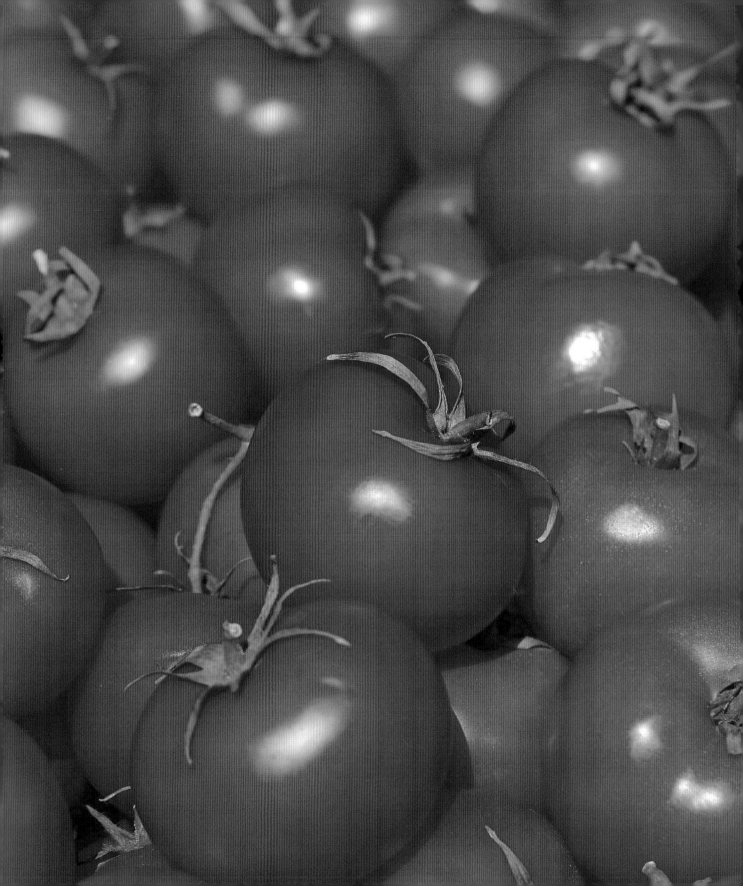

CHAPTER FOUR

FOOD AND WHAT IT DOES

food, mood and your child's behaviour

De-junking your child's diet can have a dramatic effect on his or her behaviour and moods. The food children eat affects their bodies and minds in a variety of powerful ways, so it's not surprising that their diet influences the way they behave. Food has a huge impact on your child's body, and no child feels happy when they feel peaky or below par — they want to feel healthy and full of energy. And the nutrients in food are also needed to build and maintain, and also feed, the brain.

We're not saying that certain foods will turn your child into a little angel, or make them super-brainy. But replacing the junk with nutritious foods can:

▶▶ Sustain children between meals, so they don't get hungry and grumpy.

▶▶ Balance their blood sugar levels, helping them to stay calm rather than overexcited.

▶▶ Improve their energy levels throughout the day, so they don't get tired and whiney.

▶▶ Stop them getting 'hyper' from the effects of additives.

▶▶ Help them to concentrate, and do better at school.

▶▶ Help to control ADHD (Attention Deficit Hyperactivity Disorder).

keeping them fuelled

We've already talked about how keeping children fuelled with foods that produce slow-release energy — such as wholegrains — helps to keep their blood sugar levels nice and stable. Maintaining a stable blood sugar level helps stop children from getting tired and headachy — and grumpy — when their blood sugar levels fall.

Sugary foods are bad for providing constant energy — they're quickly absorbed, but their energy is just as quickly used up, giving your child an almost instant 'energy hit', which just doesn't last.

See if you recognise this picture … Your child is hungry, and has some biscuits to keep them going until the next meal. For a little while, they feel great (though they may become overexcited). But all too soon they're hungry again – and demanding more biscuits.

Children need stable blood sugar levels in order to concentrate, so it also helps them to study at school (see Week 3 of the plan in Part 2). And many experts suggest that it's also likely that children fuelled on slow-release carbohydrates are more likely to be calm and well behaved in class, while it's those who are 'sugar fed' who are more likely to be disruptive, jumping up and down and practically bouncing off the walls.

iron deficiency

Children may develop iron deficiency if their iron intake (from their diet) doesn't keep up with their iron needs – and growing children have high iron requirements for their size. If iron deficiency isn't nipped in the bud, it can progress to anaemia.

Because iron is involved in making healthy red blood cells for carrying oxygen around the body, a lack of iron can lead to a child's body being 'hungry' for enough oxygen. This can cause a variety of symptoms.

Iron deficient children may:
▶▶ Feel tired
▶▶ Be lethargic
▶▶ Be irritable
▶▶ Have difficulty in concentrating
▶▶ Have problems remembering things

If a child isn't getting enough iron in their diet, they may feel 'not well', but be unable to explain why, so it's important to have them checked by a doctor.

You can help prevent iron deficiency by giving your child plenty of foods high in iron (see page 31). Giving them foods rich in vitamin C (such as orange juice) at the same time helps the body to take up the iron.

Even if you suspect your child may be iron deficient, *never* give him or her iron supplements except under medical supervision. Iron can build up in the body, and overdoses are dangerous and can even be fatal.

B vitamins

B vitamins are vital in releasing energy from food, but they also seem to be important in regulating our moods. Studies have found a deficiency in B vitamins to be associated with low mood and depression in adults, so it stands to reason that making sure our children get enough of these important nutrients could help them to stay happy and contented. For good sources of B vitamins, see page 30 [table of micronutrients].

additives

Food additives, especially artificial colourings, have been blamed for causing behavioural problems such as Attention Deficit Hyperactivity Disorder (ADHD). Scientists argue over just how serious the problem is, but it certainly seems that some additives cause behavioural problems in some children. Until the worst offenders in terms of chemicals are identified, we have to do a bit of detective work, and figure out whether any particular foods cause problems in our own little ones.

Here are some things to think about when you're shopping:

▶▶ Look for short ingredients lists, made up of 'real foods' you recognise.

▶▶ Buy the best quality you can afford. Cheaper ranges tend to have more additives.

▶▶ Look for foods with shorter shelf lives. It might sound a silly thing to do, but what do you think manufacturers use to extend the 'use-by date'? That's right, additives.

▶▶ Buy organic foods when you can afford it. The rules governing the additives allowed in organic ranges are far stricter than for other foods.

▶▶ Avoid luridly coloured products – few foods (except of course for fruit and vegetables) are naturally that bright. Processed foods are often coloured just to make them appeal to children.

▶▶ If there's a choice between 'plain' or 'flavoured', go for the more natural 'plain' version.

▶▶ If a product says 'free from artificial colourings' on the label, don't assume it's additive free. It could still contain artificial flavourings and preservatives.

And above all, try to make as much as possible of your family's food from scratch.

food and hyperactivity

Children's diets appear to be crucial when it comes to understanding hyperactivity. A lot of exciting research is now being carried out in this area, and many parents have found that 'de-junking' their children's diets helps to calm them down and make them less 'wild' and uncontrollable, and more 'focused' instead. The Hyperactive Children's Support Group believes that doctors should try nutrition before medication when treating children with ADHD.

We don't know how 'de-junking' helps. Could it be:

▶▶ Reducing the sugar content?

▶▶ Reducing or removing the caffeine, from cola, energy drinks and chocolate?

▶▶ Increasing the fruits and vegetables?

▶▶ Increasing the wholegrains?

▶▶ Replacing saturated and trans fats with healthier mono- and poly-unsaturated fats, especially Omega-3 essential fatty acids?

▶▶ Replacing additive-laden processed foods with wholesome home-cooked foods?

▶▶ Replacing fizzy drinks with pure water?

It's probably a combination of all of them, and different things will help different children. But does it matter what's causing the improvement, so long as it works?

food for health defence

Strong defences and a healthy immune system protect children from bugs, germs and other infections, and we can help to boost our children's immunity with food.

It's common sense that a well-nourished child is more likely to be a healthy child. A good diet will provide all the nutrients needed to maintain all of a child's various body systems, such as their brain and nervous system, their heart and lungs (the cardiovascular system), their digestive system, and their muscles and bones (the musculoskeletal system).

And diet is also critical to health through its effect on another system – the immune system. A poor diet of junk food leads to nutrient deficiencies and weakened immunity. But a healthy diet, rich in vitamins, minerals, antioxidants and phytochemicals, builds your child's natural defences against illness.

Strengthen your child's armoury against illness

Here's what you need:

▶▶ Vitamins, especially the vitamins A, C and E

▶▶ The important immune-boosting minerals – zinc and selenium

▶▶ Antioxidants and phytochemicals (such as carotenoids and anthocyanins).

Antioxidants

You've probably heard of antioxidants – an incredibly healthy group of vitamins, minerals and other micronutrients which zap harmful molecules called 'free radicals' before they can damage the body's cells.

Free radicals are everywhere. We can't escape them, as our bodies produce them naturally, and they're also in our environment. But we can bolster our children's defences against them by feeding them an antioxidant-rich diet. We can also minimise children's exposure to some forms of free radicals in the first place by avoiding deep-fried or chargrilled food and limiting their exposure to environmental pollutants such as traffic fumes and cigarette smoke. Making sure they don't get too much exposure to the sun's rays also helps.

There are many different antioxidants – these are just a few of them:

Vitamins – especially vitamin C and vitamin E

▶▶ Get vitamin A from liver, oily fish and eggs

▶▶ Get vitamin C from fruit (especially kiwifruit, strawberries and citrus fruit) and green vegetables

▶▶ Get vitamin E from nuts and seeds and their oils

Minerals – especially zinc, selenium and magnesium

▶▶ Get zinc from pumpkin seeds and sunflower seeds, shellfish, eggs and hard cheeses

▶▶ Get selenium from Brazil nuts, shellfish, kidney and liver

▶▶ Get magnesium from wholegrains, beans and lentils, and green leafy vegetables

Carotenoids

These are pigments that make fruit and vegetables yellow and orange. The body can also convert beta-carotene (one of the carotenoids) into vitamin A.

▶▶ Get carotenoids from colourful fruit and veg such as yellow and orange peppers, carrots, apricots and cantaloupe melons.

SPUDS FOR C

Perhaps surprisingly, potatoes are a good source of vitamin C, particularly if the skins are eaten. They're not as concentrated a source as fruits and green vegetables, but, because they're generally eaten in larger quantities, they make up a large proportion of most children's intake of this vitamin.

IMMUNE-BOOSTING SUPERFOODS

Blueberries

Kiwifruits

Tomatoes

Red peppers

Broccoli

Carrots

Mangoes

Sweet potatoes

Almonds

Pumpkin seeds and sunflower seeds

Anthocyanins – these pigments make fruit and vegetables red or purple.

▶▶ Get anthocyanins from blueberries, cherries and red grapes.

Fantastic Phytochemicals

Phytochemicals, or 'plant chemicals', are behind many of the healthy properties of fruit and vegetables. Some vitamins (those found in vegetarian sources) are phytochemicals, but there are plenty more, such as:

▶▶ The pigments that make tomatoes red, carrots orange and broccoli green.

▶▶ The substances that gives onions their characteristic smell and eye-watering properties.

▶▶ The chemicals that give raw Brussels sprouts their mouth-puckering taste.

It's easy to pack your child's diet with fantastic phytochemicals – just give them plenty of fruit and veg!

food for a healthy digestive system

All the nutritious food in the world isn't going to benefit our children if they can't digest and absorb it properly, and, for that, they need a healthy digestive system.

Put simply, your child's digestive system is a food processor, taking in food, chopping it up and breaking it down, so that it can be absorbed and used by the body. Digestion begins in the mouth, when food is chewed and swallowed, and continues in the stomach, and then further down in the intestines. As soon as the food is broken down into simple enough molecules, it is absorbed into the bloodstream and used by the body.

There are some foods that help keep a child's digestive system working healthily. Other foods, however, make life difficult for the gut.

And it's no surprise that it's the healthy wholefoods that promote a happy digestive system, and the junk food that makes it hard for the digestive system to function at its best.

Tummy troubles

A healthy diet can go a long way towards preventing tummy problems and, if your child follows our 6-Week Junk-Free Plan, you'll almost certainly find that they suffer less from diarrhoea and constipation.

Diarrhoea

Diarrhoea occurs when the body doesn't absorb enough water from the waste products in the digestive system – and, unfortunately, watery waste equals 'the runs'! It generally occurs due to an infection ('tummy bug'), or if the gut is irritated, but it can also be brought on by emotional upsets.

Don't worry if your child doesn't feel like eating if they're suffering from diarrhoea – it's much more important to keep children hydrated with plenty of water, as they'll be losing extra fluids.

Once they feel like food again, offer them things like a dry cracker or a rice cake, some dry toast, or plain boiled rice, until their digestive system is up to taking less bland food. Avoid dairy foods until their digestion is completely back to normal, as even children who generally have no problems with dairy may become slightly intolerant to it after a bout of tummy trouble.

You can help prevent diarrhoea by giving your child foods rich in fibre, as this absorbs water and 'bulks up' the food waste.

Good sources of fibre include:

▶▶ Wholegrains – wholemeal bread, brown rice, wholemeal pasta, bulgur, buckwheat, oats

▶▶ Beans and lentils

▶▶ Fruit and vegetables (especially if the skins are eaten)

> **Don't be tempted to suddenly increase the fibre in your child's diet – ironically, this can actually cause diarrhoea or constipation. Instead, gradually increase the amount of fibre in your child's meals and snacks, to allow the digestive system to adapt and get used to the change. This will also allow you to see if the extra fibre is filling them up too much – if they start getting full up before they've finished, you could be overdoing it.**

Constipation

Constipation can make children feel truly miserable, yet they may be too embarrassed to tell you about the problem. Alternatively, a child may not realise what's wrong – they just feel really uncomfortable.

Inadequate hydration is the main cause of constipation, so encourage children to have regular drinks, preferably of pure water.

Another common cause of constipation is not enough fibre in the diet. Food moves along the digestive system by means of muscular contractions – rather like squeezing goo along a flexible rubber tube! The digestive system finds it easier to squeeze if it has plenty of bulk to work on, and that's where fibre comes in yet again.

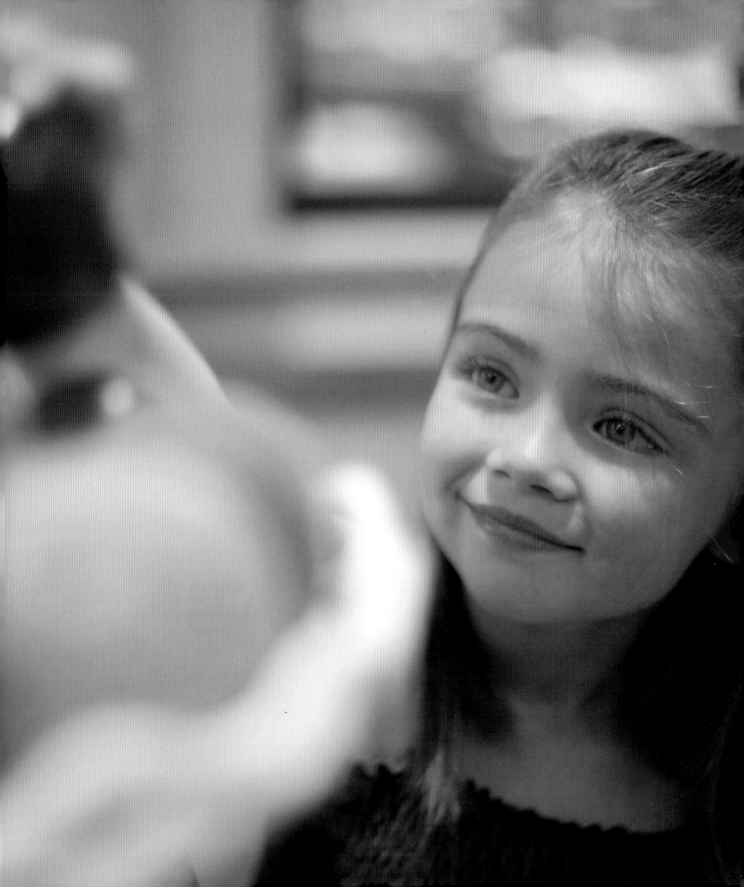

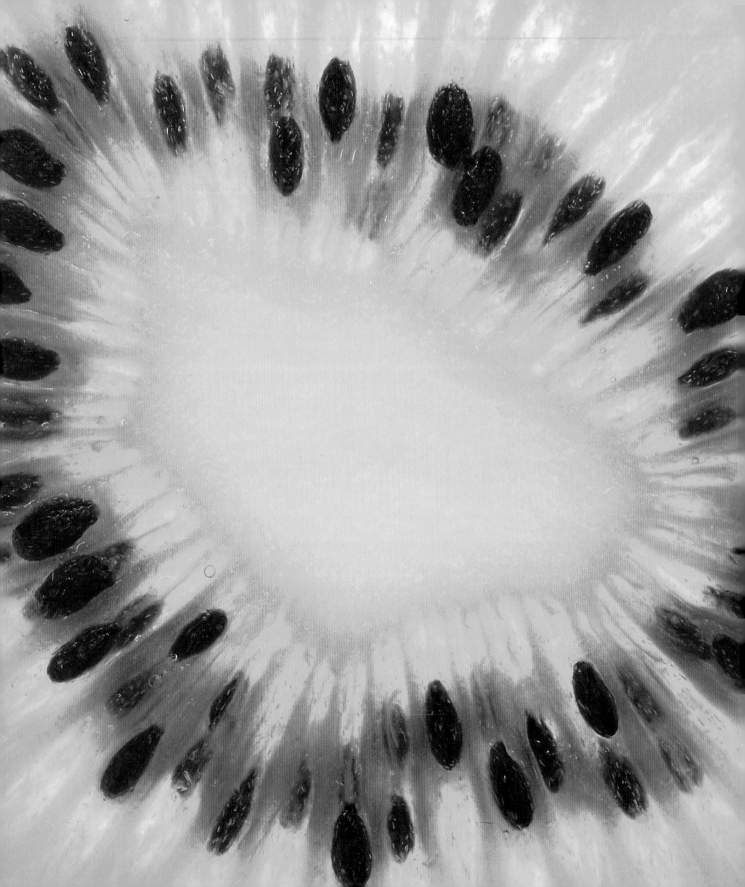

CHAPTER FIVE

PERSUADING CHILDREN

It's sad but true – given a choice of what to eat, the vast majority of children will choose the unhealthy option. They'd rather have cola than water, would prefer chips to a jacket potato, and an apple would come a poor second to a bag of sweets.

This generation of children has grown up surrounded by salty, sugary, fatty and luridly coloured food. And, if that's what we let them get used to, anything else will taste bland, or be 'sour', or boring – initially, at least.

Unfortunately, if left to their own devices, a child with a sweet tooth will grow up to be an adult with a sweet tooth. Or, most likely, an adult with very few of their own teeth! And, if a child develops a daily 'crisp habit', that taste is likely to stay with them for life.

But, even if they already have some bad habits, these can be changed – you just have to do it gradually, sometimes sneakily, and never too blatantly!

Children who eat healthily during their primary school and 'tweenage' years are more likely to enjoy good health when they're adolescents and young adults. And by this time they're old enough to realise, 'Hang on, when I eat healthily, I feel full of energy and can enjoy life. But when I pig out on junk food, I feel stodgy, lethargic and put on weight.'

But are children's food choices all a matter of 'taste'? Do they choose the less healthy food solely because it's 'yummy'.

Apparently not.

Although children say they like the foods they do solely because they taste nice, their choices are also being guided by a subtle web of influences.

what do children think children eat?

It sounds a strange question, doesn't it? But children seem to have very firm ideas of what 'real' children eat. In a fascinating study commissioned by Barnados, children were asked this question. The resounding answer was … 'children eat fast food'.

And when shown a picture of a junk food meal and a healthy meal, they said that children were far more likely to eat the burger and chips. That was described as 'yum'.

not wanting to be different

No child wants to be 'different'. If everyone else is eating junk food, how many children will stick their necks out to choose a healthy option? It takes a very self-confident child to hand over his pocket money for an apple in a shop when all his friends are buying sweets or crisps.

And, sadly, it's all too easy for a child to be embarrassed if you send them to school with a healthy wholemeal pasta salad, a natural yoghurt with honey and sunflower seeds, and a crispy apple. When their friends' lunchboxes contain white-bread sandwiches, crisps and a snack-size chocolate bar, they may fear being ridiculed.

wanting to be part of the 'in crowd'

Advertisers call it 'peer-to-peer' selling, and it's based on the 'herd mentality'. If a particular flavour of crisps becomes popular and fashionable in a school, that's what everyone will want to bring in their lunchbox. And if the most popular girl in the class always chooses a particular kind of fizzy drink, well, that's obviously the best, isn't it?

advertising

Although, deep down, most children know that advertising is all about trying to sell them something, they still seem to view TV advertisements as an 'information channel', useful for telling them about all the yummy new foods out there. 'Yummy', in their opinion, but almost always unhealthy. Studies have shown that most food advertising aimed at children is for sugary breakfast cereals, sweets and chocolate, savoury snacks such as crisps, and fast-food outlets. And do the healthier options get a look in? Not a bit of it. When did you last see an advertisement telling children that fish, apples or lentils were fab?

Advertisers are clever – they sell to children using fun themes, rather than by saying it's 'good for them'. And in many cases, they *couldn't* claim the food was good for them.

Advertising also plays to the children's idea that it's good to eat what their friends are eating. While adverts targeting adults often feature them relaxing alone with this luxury ice cream or that indulgent hot chocolate, a food manufacturer who wants to appeal to children is more likely to choose a very different approach. It appears that adverts aimed at children are more likely to show groups of happy children having fun and enjoying the food – together! The subliminal message? 'Me and all my friends eat the same thing.' And yet another reason for children to want to eat manufactured processed food, rather than the homemade or natural alternative.

So what can you do? The first thing to realise is that advertising is designed to sell more of the product and enable the manufacturer to gain an advantage over their competitors. Your best defence against this kind of onslaught is to learn to read the labels and make your own decision on whether the product is something you want your child to eat. If it isn't, don't buy it – you have the final say!

▶▶ Make time to watch TV advertising directed at children so that you are aware of the messages they are receiving.

▶▶ As far as possible, try to limit their TV watching to programmes without advertising.

▶▶ Remember, it's not only children who are being targeted by advertising. Parents are bombarded by flashes declaring 'added calcium' and 'fortified with vitamins'. But the amounts of these added nutrients can be very small indeed, and nowhere does the packaging list all of the valuable nutrients that have been lost in the processing. Again, the message is 'fresh is best'.

children's food and other gimmicks

Once upon a time, there was no such thing as 'children's food'. Little people simply ate smaller portions of big people's foods.

Now, however, the manufacturers have jumped on the 'children's food' bandwagon, and it seems that, in order to appeal to children, food has to be 'child sized' and

individually wrapped. Or formed into little shapes and coated in orange breadcrumbs, dipped into little pots of sauce, or branded with the latest popular cartoon character.

Think of all the 'lunchbox' ranges you see at the supermarket – all designed to appeal to children, not to mention busy parents! And it's no crime to use them as a time-saver every now and then. But it's almost as easy to cut a large block of cheese into matchbox-sized pieces and wrap them in cling film for the week's lunchboxes, than to pick up individually wrapped cheese portions especially for lunchboxes. Almost as easy – and certainly cheaper! And what are you paying for? Some fancy packaging and other marketing tricks.

Fortunately, some manufacturers are developing a sense of responsibility. They're reducing the fat, sugar and salt levels in their 'children's ranges'. But the fact that children's ranges exist still remains – making it that little bit more difficult to persuade our youngsters to eat good home-cooked fare. Difficult, but not impossible – we'll show you how. Homemade food can be just as exciting as the latest children's cartoon-character spaghetti shape in tomato sauce!

brand awareness

Children are alarmingly brand aware, and research has shown that most will choose a 'commercial brand' of a food such as a chocolate bar rather than a supermarket's own brand. This is especially true if they're going to be eating the food in front of their friends.

Brand awareness makes it more difficult to persuade children to eat 'unbranded' foods that you've made from scratch. You have to make it appeal in different ways.

help – what can I do?

First of all, don't panic! If your child sees that refusing the foods you want them to eat, and demanding the things you disapprove of gets a reaction – any reaction – they'll carry on doing it. Just for the attention – it's a power thing. Children don't realise they're using this kind of psychology, but it's powerful stuff, as any stressed-out parent who desperately struggles to try to get at least *something* that's healthy inside their child will agree. If junior digs in his heels and seems intent on staging a one-child dietary revolution, most parents will worry – it's a natural reaction.

Getting children on side

Making healthy food trendy may look like an uphill battle – but that's no reason not to attempt it. Plenty of schools are trying this technique, and finding that, once one child tries and likes something, it's much easier to get their friends to follow suit.

You need to make healthy food FUN – and that's what this book is all about.

Tasting times

If you're introducing something new, let the child try just a little and explain that they only need to have one taste. If you put a large spoonful on their plate and they think they have to eat it all, they're more likely to dig their heels in and decide they won't like it, before the fork gets anywhere near their mouth. If they absolutely don't want to taste it, just try again another day. Forcing the issue is a sure-fire way of turning mealtimes into battlegrounds and making a child hate that food for years to come.

Where it's practical, allow children to serve themselves, so that they choose how much to put on their plates. Research has shown that children who are allowed to choose actually eat more and may be more adventurous about trying new foods.

Don't be tempted to urge children to eat 'just one more mouthful', then 'just another' over and over again, or to clean their plate. Scientists have found that children are better than adults are at judging when they have eaten enough. If your child feels full, prompting them to eat more can disrupt their sense of satiety and could lead to habitual overeating. It can also put them off that particular food, and you would not want to encourage either of these things.

And never use food as a bribe or a reward! If you want to reward your child, give them something totally unrelated to food, such as a trip to the cinema or a book.

Presentation pays

It really is true that to a certain extent we eat with our eyes – and children are no different. If their meal looks like a mountain of mush or they're faced with a pale and anaemic-looking lump of steamed or baked chicken, they're more likely to turn up their little noses than if their food looks colourful and appetising. For example, slice chicken breasts and reconstruct them. You can also give them colour and flavour by dusting with a little Cajun or Jamaican jerk seasoning before baking.

Feeding 'fussy' eaters

Children are entitled to have likes and dislikes, and even a few foods they just can't stomach, but some children become fussy in the extreme. Sometimes fussy eating can be due to the child (whether consciously or unconsciously) exerting their independence and seeing how far they can push the boundaries.

Trying to feed a fussy eater is extremely frustrating, and picky eating can lead to a child's diet becoming unbalanced. This makes it important to try to nip the problem in the bud.

Make sure that you don't prejudice their food choices with your own likes and dislikes. Just because you can't abide tomatoes or olives, that's no reason why they should feel the same way.

Don't label your child. If they hear you describing them as a 'fussy eater' or 'difficult to feed', they'll quickly realise they have gained the attention they may be seeking. Instead, praise them when they do eat, or try a new food.

And don't give up if you try a new food and they refuse it – try again with that food about a week later, perhaps cooked or presented slightly differently, as it can take many attempts before a child likes a new taste. Don't make a big performance out of producing the new food; it should just appear on the table with everything else. If your child points out that they've had it before and didn't like it, just raise your eyebrows and say, 'Didn't you? Well, perhaps you could give it another try – it's a bit different this time.'

If your child has tried the food ten times or so, and still 'hates it', you'll probably have to accept that this isn't a battle worth fighting. Try to get those nutrients into your child with other foods.

Also, children (and adults) may suddenly change their food preferences, often after years of disliking something. A 'tomato-hater', for example, may suddenly decide many years in the future that they love them, when their girlfriend or boyfriend cooks with them, or when they go away to college.

▶▶ Only introduce one new food at a time.
▶▶ Serve food at 'child-friendly' temperatures. If the food is too hot, they may burn their lips or mouth. Also, waiting for food to cool down before they can eat it gives them time to think of reasons why they shouldn't eat it.
▶▶ Children will often eat what they see their friends eating, so invite 'good eaters' round for tea.
▶▶ If you child refuses a meal, don't be tempted to increase the size or number of snacks to fill the gap. If you stick to your guns, the chances are they will be hungry at the next mealtime.

If you really are concerned about your child's picky eating, seek professional advice.

DON'T SAY THIS:
'You're not leaving the table until you eat those peas!'
SAY THIS:
'Just try one mouthful.'

Forcing children to clear their plate can weaken their ability to detect when they're full. It's also not good for your relationship with your child, and can set up bad attitudes towards food.

DON'T SAY THIS:
'You're just being difficult – eat those carrots!'
SAY THIS:
'What is it that you don't like about those carrots?'

It might just be the way you've cooked the food that they dislike.

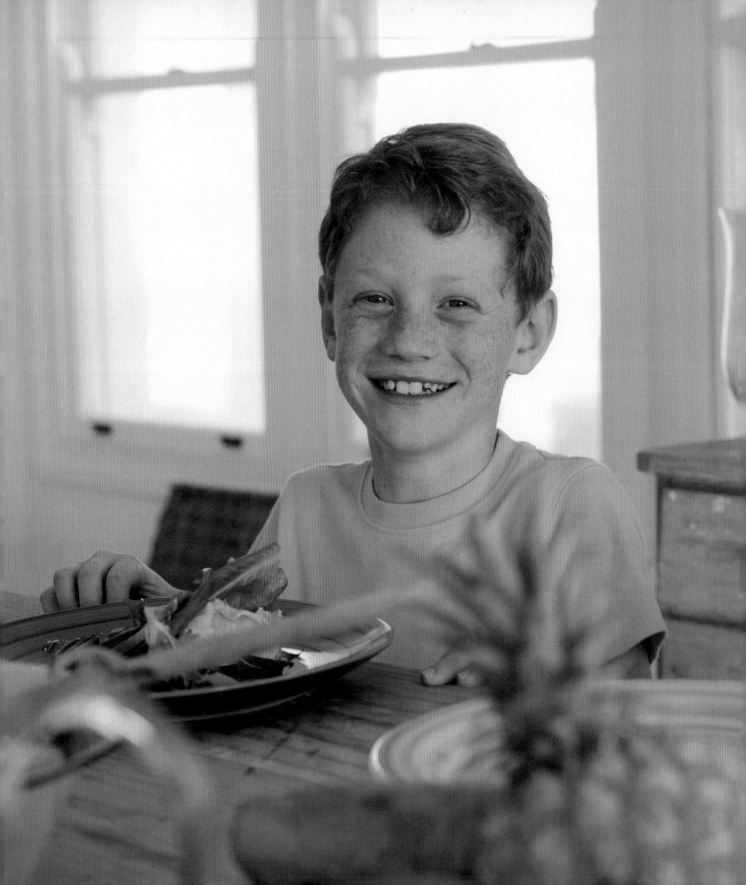

PART 2
THE 6-WEEK JUNK-FREE EATING PLAN

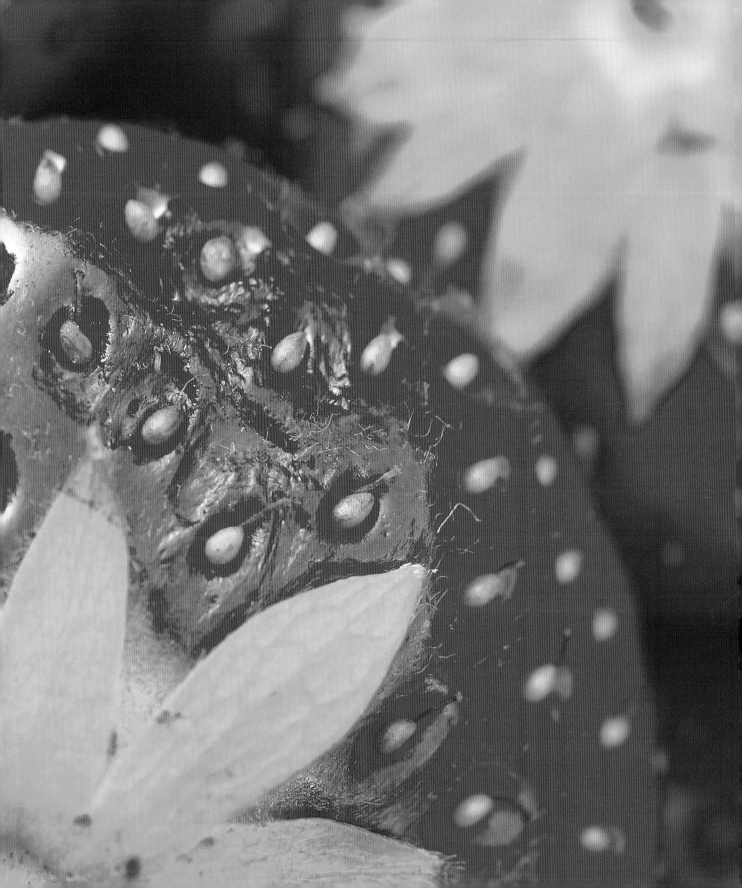

CHAPTER SIX

INTRODUCTION TO THE 6-WEEK JUNK-FREE PLAN

Now you're ready to start the 6-Week Junk-Free Plan. The plan is nothing to be scared of – it starts off very gently and builds up over the six weeks. And once you get going, you'll quickly begin to see the benefits.

Each week you'll concentrate on a different area of your child's – and your family's – diet so by the end of week 6 the new way of eating will be second nature to you all.

WEEK 1: De-junk your **storecupboard**, phasing out the less-healthy foods and gradually replacing them with more nutritious alternatives.

WEEK 2: Learn to be a smart, **healthy shopper** – tips to help you decipher the labels, make healthy choices, and resist pester power.

WEEK 3: Find out why the first meal of the day is so important, and set your child up for the day with our power-packed **breakfasts**.

WEEK 4: Learn what makes up a really good **lunch**, then try our 'Pick and Mix' lunchboxes, and simple, healthy weekend and holiday meals.

WEEK 5: Enjoy the benefits of a tasty family **dinner**, with our satisfying recipes featuring different food groups on different days, to help ensure you all get a balanced diet.

WEEK 6: Discover the wonders of **snacks**, and help sustain your child between mealtimes and top up their nutrient levels.

It's a very **positive** plan.

▶▶ It concentrates on the benefits of fresh healthy food, rather than the negatives of unhealthy food.

▶▶ It highlights the exciting new foods you can add to your child's diet, rather than the foods you're going to be cutting down or out.

▶▶ It helps you take control, making your own healthy meals, rather than getting depressed or angry at the amount of unhealthy additives in processed foods.

Don't sweat the small stuff! You're doing great, simply by caring enough about your child's present and future health to have picked up this book and resolved to change things.

Celebrate the progress you're making in improving your child's diet, rather than dwelling on the lapses – and there will be 'wobbles' and 'off days'. There will be times when the plan unravels. Don't panic – it's not the end of the world. Just keep at it, and recognise your successes as you go.

It's also important that your child knows that you recognise that they are *their* successes, too. Praise them when they make the right choices or try something new.

It may be called the 'Junk-Free' Plan, but make sure your child knows it's not all about laying down the law and removing all of the things they think are nice to eat.

Remember, we're not even going to attempt to get your family 100% 'Junk Free'. That's not realistic. No one can get it 'right' 100% of the time – and you shouldn't even try. It's all about balance and moderation.

I would never ban my child from eating junk food as this simply makes it even more desirable. There's nothing wrong with them having a chocolate biscuit or chicken nuggets now and again.

In fact, those poor kids put on ultra-strict diets by their fanatical mums and dads are more likely to rush straight to my secret stash of goodies, and stick their heads in the biscuit tin trying to cram as much forbidden chocolate biscuits down their throats as possible.

Just do the best you can. Every little bit of progress is just that – Progress!

In Part 3, we'll spend some more time exploring how to maintain a 'de-junked' lifestyle. And you'll be pleased to see that it's not condemning you to a lifestyle of austerity and no more treats!

Instead, it's all about developing your child's interest in healthy eating, getting them involved, and helping them to 'connect' with their food.

You'll find all of these children's favourites in the plan, but they've all been *healthified*!

Chicken nuggets (see Chicken Dippers)

Beefburgers (see Homemade Beefburgers, plus Chicken, Turkey and Bean Burgers)

Chips (see Chunky Chips)

Potato wedges

Pizza (see Muffin Chicken Pizza)

Fish fingers (see Homemade Fish Fingers)

Milk shake (see Nectarine and Banana Milk shake)

Muffins (see Fast Fruity Muffins)

You may want to skip ahead and have a quick read through, but it's not essential, and it's totally up to you.

Otherwise, simply dive in to the 6-Week Junk-Free Plan – you've nothing to lose, and everything to gain.

It's all about common sense and all things in moderation!

getting started

Before we embark on revamping your child's diet, let's take a look at what they're eating right now.

The results may surprise you – it's all too easy to let unhealthy foods sneak into your child's day. But knowing where you're starting from will allow you to see how much progress you're making through the coming weeks.

And even if you find that your child's diet is pretty good already, there will probably be some troublesome little areas that could do with taking a look at.

Sit down and do the quiz, then work out your scores for Junk Points and Health Points.

take the quiz

Junk points

General questions

☐ Does your child add salt to food at the table? (score 1 Junk Point if the answer is yes)

Questions about how many times in the last week your child ate something

☐ How many times in the last week did your child have deep fried chips – not baked oven chips? (score 1 Junk Point for each portion)

☐ How many times in the last week did your child have deep fried foods – not including chips? (score 1 Junk Point for each time)

☐ How many times in the last week did your child eat at a fast food restaurant? (score 1 Junk Point for each time)

☐ How many times in the last week did your child skip a meal? (score 1 Junk Point for every skipped meal)

☐ How many times in the last week did your child eat a takeaway meal? (score 1 Junk Point for each meal)

☐ How many times in the last week did your child eat processed meat products such as sausages, burgers or nuggets? (score 1 Junk Point for each time)

☐ How many chocolate bars did your child have in the last week? (score 2 Junk Points for each bar)

☐ How many packets of sweets (a small packet or the equivalent) did your child have in the last week? (score 1 Junk Point for each packet)

☐ How many cakes and biscuits did your child eat in the last week, not including 'healthy' low-fat, low-sugar versions you made yourself? (score 1 Junk Point for each cake or biscuit)

Questions about how many times a day your child eats something

☐ How many cans or glasses of fizzy drink does your child have in an average day? (score 1 Junk Point for each can or glass)

☐ How many caffeine-containing foods or drinks (cola, energy drinks, tea, coffee, chocolate) does your child have in an average day? (score 1 Junk Point for each serving)

☐ How many packets of crisps or other salty snacks does your child have in an average day? (score 1 Junk Point for each packet)

Health points

General questions

☐ Does your child always eat breakfast? (score 1 Health Point if they always eat breakfast and 2 Health Points if it's always a healthy breakfast)

☐ Does your child drink the recommended 8–10 glasses of water every day? (score 2 Health Points if the answer is yes)

☐ Does your child eat some nuts or seeds every day? (score 1 Health Point if the answer is yes)

Questions about how many times in the last week your child ate something

☐ How many times in the last week did your child eat fish? (score 1 Health Point for each serving)

☐ How many times in the last week did your child eat oily fish such as salmon, mackerel or sardines? (score 1 Health Point for each serving, on top of any points from the previous question)

☐ How many times in the last week did your child eat beans or lentils? (score 1 Health Point for each serving)

Questions about how many times a day your child eats something

☐ How many portions of fruit does your child eat in an average day? (score 1 Health Point for each portion)

☐ How many portions of vegetables does your child eat in an average day? (score 1 Health Point for each portion)

☐ On an average day, how many portions of calcium rich food does your child have? Calcium foods include dairy products, tinned salmon or sardines with the bones, sesame seeds, green leafy vegetables. (score 1 Health Point for each portion)

Scoring

In an ideal world, every child would score zero Junk Points, with a Health Points score in the twenties.

But there's nothing wrong with occasional indulgences of chocolate, cake and the like, so long as they're only a very small part of your child's diet.

Concentrate instead on increasing those Health Points! Children are far more inclined to respond to healthy-eating messages if you stress the positive.

If your child enjoys the quiz, repeat it every week or two through the 6-Week Junk-Free Plan. If you start off with a Junk Points score higher than your Health Points, see how quickly you can make those Health Points overtake the Junk! Then concentrate on increasing the difference between the two.

As you work your way through the 6-Week Junk-Free Plan, talk to your child about how you're going to increase those Health Points.

▶▶ 'You had a healthy breakfast every day – that's another 2 Health Points'

▶▶ 'We're having beans tonight – that's another Health Point'

▶▶ 'How many pieces of fruit did you eat today? Three? That's 3 more Health Points.'

▶▶ 'There are some pumpkin seeds in your lunchbox, so that's another Health Point for your chart.'

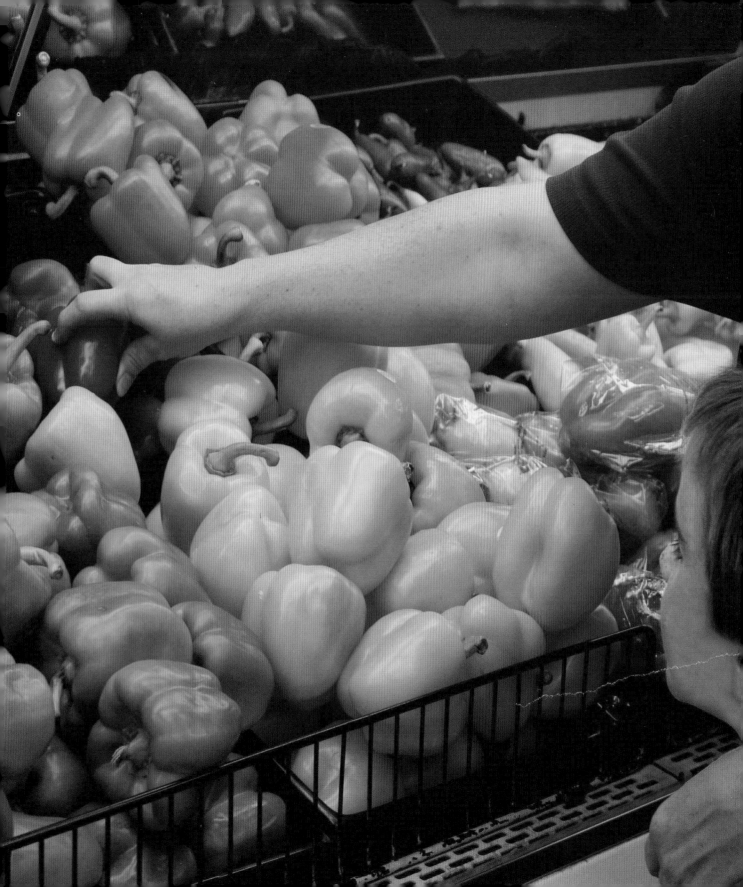

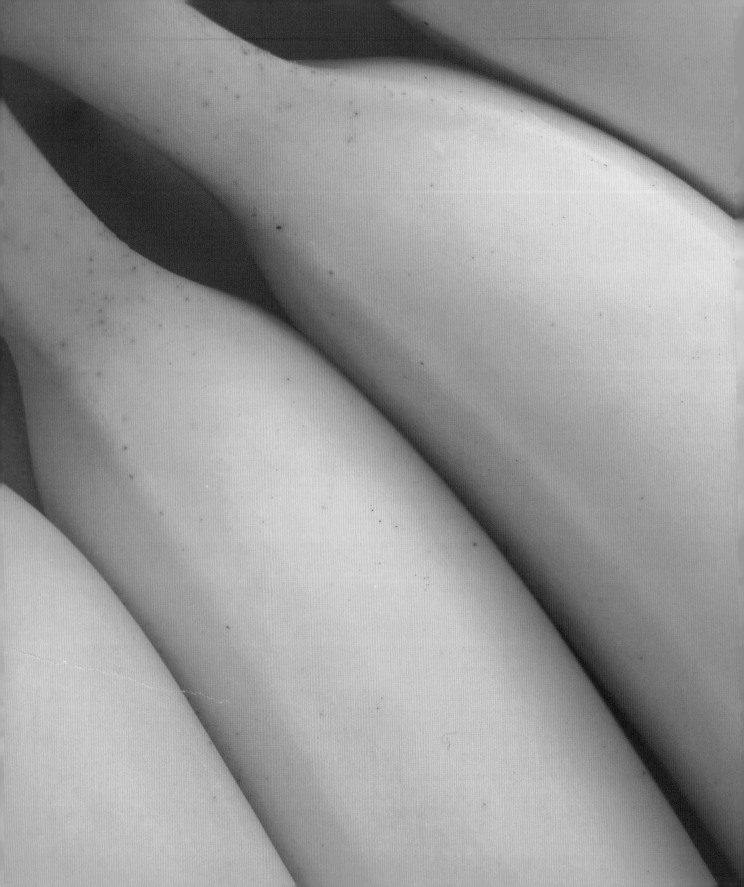

CHAPTER SEVEN

THE 6-WEEK JUNK-FREE EATING PLAN

starting the plan

You're now ready to start the 6-Week Junk-Free Eating Plan. But don't panic. Like I said before, the plan is very gentle and will introduce you slowly to the principles of healthy eating. In fact, the first two weeks are more about 'learning' – how to find healthy alternatives to food you may already eat, and how to make sense of all that bewildering information we're faced with at the supermarket – than 'doing'.

The great thing about this plan is that you and your child won't feel like you're following a plan at all! Because you ease yourself in gently, by gradually making simple healthy substitutions and by learning how to decipher food labels,

you'll be learning new habits and eating healthily before you even realise!

This plan is all about flexibility – you can adapt it to your own family's tastes and preferences, and the fact that it encourages your child's involvement means there's a great chance they'll develop an interest in food you'd never have thought was possible.

So, turn the page, and look forward to a healthy junk-free future – for you and your child.

WEEK 1 – DE-JUNK YOUR KITCHEN

The first step is to get rid of the less than healthy food in your kitchen. But don't worry, it's a gradual and painless process. It doesn't involve any wasteful throwing away of food, or buying lots of expensive and exotic foods.

Just follow these guidelines and, before you know it, your home will be all but junk-free, and your family's health will be reaping the benefits.

healthy alternatives

Every time you run out of an 'unhealthy' food, replace it with a healthier alternative.

▶▶ When you run out of 'standard' tomato ketchup, replace it with a low-salt, low-sugar version.

▶▶ Replace 'standard' baked beans and tinned spaghetti with those that are reduced in salt and sugar.

▶▶ Replace 'standard' salad cream and mayonnaise with low-fat.

▶▶ Replace salted peanuts with unsalted peanuts roasted in their shells, or other unsalted nuts.

▶▶ Replace highly sweetened breakfast cereals with plain wholegrain versions, such as porridge oats, unsweetened muesli or wholewheat bisks.

▶▶ Start buying natural yoghurt for livening up with healthy extras instead of brightly coloured and sweetened 'children's yoghurts'.

▶▶ Buy pure fruit juice instead of squash or fizzy drinks.

inspiring suggestions

We're not going to ask you to stock up on a huge list of new ingredients that your family might not even like. Just add one new food to your shopping list every week, to give it a try.

Here are just a few ideas:

▶▶ Try a new grain, such as bulgur wheat, couscous, buckwheat or millet.

▶▶ If you've always had 'white' pasta and rice before, give the brown versions a try.

▶▶ Try a nut or seed you haven't had before.

▶▶ Try a new herb or spice – how about tarragon, dill, or lemon grass?

▶▶ Pick up a tin of pulses, such as borlotti beans, chick peas, red kidney beans or tinned lentils.

▶▶ Try tahini – a delicious and nutritious sesame seed paste.

▶▶ Prowl the fresh fruit section of your local supermarket or greengrocer, and try some of the more exotic fresh produce, such as kiwifruit, Sharon fruit, blueberries or pomegranates.

▶▶ Or how about some more unusual vegetables, such as sweet potatoes, pak choi or beansprouts?

We need to go back to basics and not be so reliant on those expensive ready meals. They can be very convenient, but nothing beats good home-cooked food.

the healthy storecupboard

With a well-stocked storecupboard, you can rustle up tasty meals in no time. Don't be daunted by the length of the list below – the foods are just suggestions.

Grains

Rice

Oats

Millet

Couscous

Nuts

Almonds

Brazil nuts

Cashew nuts

Hazelnuts

Walnuts

Seeds

Pumpkin seeds

Sesame seeds

Sunflower seeds

Pulses (tinned or dried)

Cannellini beans (tinned)

Red kidney beans (tinned)

Chick peas (tinned or dried)

Red lentils (dried)

Continental lentils (tinned or dried)

Dried fruit

Raisins/sultanas/currants

Dried apricots (unsulphured and natural)

Dried figs

Flour

Wholewheat plain and self-raising flour

White plain and self-raising flour

Strong bread flour

Tins

Tomatoes

Fish (salmon, sardines, mackerel, tuna)

Fruit in natural juice

Sweetcorn (low-sugar, low-salt)

Baked beans (low-sugar, low-salt)

Rice pudding (low-fat)

Long-life cartons

Pure fruit juice

Long-life semi-skimmed or skimmed milk

Long-life non-dairy 'milk' such as soya milk or rice milk

Herbs and spices

Mixed herbs/spices

Basil

Mint

Ground ginger

Cinnamon

Curry powder

Miscellaneous

Stock cubes (low-salt) or bouillon powder

Tomato puree

Soy sauce (low-salt)

Mustard

WEEK 2 – SMART SHOPPING

I was very lucky when I was growing up because my mum was a good, old-fashioned cook, who prepared everything from scratch and shopped for that night's food every day. There were no big superstores with massive chilled counters selling microwave meals or expensive kids' lunchboxes full of fat and additives. She would go to the butchers, the fishmongers, the bakers and the greengrocers, buying just what she needed. Everything she bought would be seasonal.

However, if you're like most parents, you probably do your main shop at the supermarket and your time is limited, but you still want to make the best choices. You need to be able to see through the clever ruses put in your path by canny manufacturers, all keen for you to buy their less-than-healthy products. But added to that, you might face pressure from the Mini Mafia who may be shopping with you, pestering for the breakfast cereal advertised by their favourite cartoon character or TV star, or the sweets that 'everyone else at school' eats.

Follow these tips to stay on the nutritional straight and narrow when you're at the supermarket:

▶▶ Plan the week's menus, right down to snacks. You can stay a little bit flexible, but it's good to know you've got something for every day of the week. And you'll be less likely to buy things 'just in case we need some of that'.

▶▶ Make a detailed list – and stick to it! This is particularly important if your budget is tight, but leave a little leeway so that you can take advantage of new season's fresh produce as it comes on to the supermarket shelves, as well as buy one get one free offers, and four items for the price of three (particularly useful when it comes to fresh fruit and vegetables).

▶▶ Learn the layout of your supermarket, and only visit the aisles you need to. In other words, spend your time in fresh fruit and veg, and skip the fizzy drinks aisle. You'll save time too!

▶▶ Never go shopping when you're hungry or tired – you're more likely to give in to temptation.

▶▶ Order your shopping online – you're less likely to succumb to impulse buys, as you won't walk past all those tempting items on the shelves. You also won't have to contend with pester power!

▶▶ Look into ordering an organic 'fruit and vegetable box' from a local farm or a national company.

learning to use the labels

Food labels are meant to help us to make healthy choices by informing us what we're eating, but they can be more confusing than helpful.

Manufacturers obviously want us to buy their products, so they make a point of shouting their health benefits from the rooftops, often in the form of banners, slogans and healthy claims on the packaging.

But some of these claims are misleading in the extreme.

For a long time, it's been very difficult to decide how 'healthy' a product was, because the laws governing health claims on packaging weren't terribly consistent. Now, new laws are being introduced by the European Union, to tighten up the loopholes and create a level playing field for products sold in all EU countries.

UNDERSTANDING THE HEALTH CLAIMS

Low calorie:
No more than 40 kcal per 100g for foods, and 20 kcal per 100ml for drinks.

Reduced-calorie, fat or sugar:
30% fewer calories, fat or sugar than the 'standard' version.

Calorie-free:
No more than 4 kcal per 100 ml (there are different rules for artificial sweeteners).

Fat-free:
No more than 0.5g fat per 100g or 100ml.

Sugar-free:
No more than 0.5g sugars per 100g or 100ml.

Low-sodium/Low-salt:
No more than 0.12g sodium per 100g or 100ml, no more than 0.3g salt per 100g or 100ml.

High-fibre:
Must contain at least 6g fibre per 100g OR at least 3g fibre per 100kcal.

At the time of writing, manufacturers were being given until 2009 to abide by all of the new regulations, so expect them to be phased in over that time.

Is it High or Low In ...?
The Food Standards Agency has produced some helpful guidelines on whether the amount of a nutrient in a food is 'a lot' or 'a little'.

Amount of nutrient per serving	This is a lot	This is a little
Total fat	20g or more	3g or less
Saturated fat	5g or more	1g or less
Sugars	10g or more	2g or less
Fibre	3g or more	0.5g or less
Sodium	0.5g or more	0.1g or less
Salt	1.25g or more	0.25g or less

Remember that ingredients are listed in order of how much the product contains.

Stop or Go at the Traffic Lights
'Traffic light' labelling on food packaging provides an at-a-glance way of deciding on whether a food fits into your healthy-eating plan.

They're designed to show you whether the food is high (red light), medium (amber light) or low (green light) in potentially harmful fat, saturated fat, salt and sugar.

For example, if you see one or more red lights on the packaging, you know that food is high in something that's not good for you.

Red = high in unhealthy substance – eat only occasionally

Amber = medium in unhealthy substance – eat some of the time

Green = low in unhealthy substance – eat most of the time

So, just because a food has one or more red lights, it doesn't mean you can't eat it as part of a healthy diet – you just need to limit it to only occasionally.

How traffic lights help:

▶▶ They give you an idea of the overall 'healthiness' of a product – the more green lights, the better

▶▶ They can help stop you overshooting your recommended limits for the nutritional 'baddies'. If, for example, you're having a lunch with a 'red light' for salt (ie, it's high in salt), you can take special care that the other products you buy have green lights for salt.

▶▶ They help you choose between similar products. If, for example, you're choosing between two tomato ketchups, you can go for the one with the most green lights and the fewest reds. You can also see which has the 'best' colour light for salt or sugar, if these are of particular concern for you and your family.

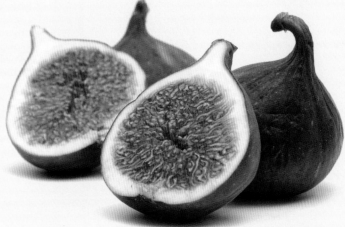

WEEK 3 – BREAKFAST

kick start the day

A healthy breakfast really *does* set you up for a good day – and this is especially true for children.

A healthy breakfast helps keep children's blood sugar levels balanced through the morning, so they're less likely to be irritable and troublesome in class. They're also more alert, and find it easier to concentrate on their lessons.

My friend who is a teacher says she can always tell the little ones who don't get a decent breakfast because they can't pay attention and sometimes even fall asleep in class. A good breakfast is vital for everyone, but especially for youngsters, and is not only important for their health but will make them better at their lessons.

A nourishing breakfast also makes it easier for children to meet their nutrient requirements for the day. Missing breakfast makes it much harder to make up the 'lost' nutrients later in the day.

> **All of the breakfasts in our 6-Week Junk-Free Plan include these three elements:**
>
> - **Fruit – for vitamins, and to start your child on their way to 'five-a-day'.**
> - **A slow-release carbohydrate – for sustained energy.**
> - **A calcium-rich dairy food (milk or yoghurt) – for building healthy bones and teeth, and to provide body-building, sustaining protein.**

the junk-free breakfast plan

Every day, choose any breakfast from this list. Try to have at least three different breakfasts each week. Different foods contain different nutrients, so by eating a variety of nutritious foods, your child maximises their chance of getting all the nutrients they need.

Egg on toast

▶▶ A banana.

▶▶ Slice of toast topped with a poached or scrambled egg.

▶▶ Small glass of milk.

Porridge or cereal

▶▶ An apple cut into wedges, or ½ glass pure fruit juice topped up with ½ glass water.

▶▶ A bowl of porridge or low sugar cereal (go for ones like Wheat bisks, bran flakes, shredded wheat or puffed wheat) with semi-skimmed milk.

▶▶ Slice of toast with low-fat spread and honey, marmalade, jam or peanut butter.

Beans on toast

▶▶ A banana.

▶▶ Slice of toast topped with 3 tablespoons of reduced-sugar, reduced-salt baked beans.

▶▶ Small glass of milk.

Peanut butter on toast

▶▶ An apple cut into wedges.

▶▶ 2 slices wholemeal toast with peanut butter, low sugar jam or cottage cheese with pineapple.

▶▶ Small glass of milk.

Fruit bowl

▶▶ ½ glass pure fruit juice topped up with ½ glass water.

▶▶ Bowl of fruit – a chopped banana, apple and ½ mango – topped with a plain yoghurt, a drizzle of honey and 2 tablespoons of no-sugar muesli or a tablespoon of chopped nuts.

Pancakes

These pancakes are great to make at the weekend. Cook enough for a few days and keep them in the freezer.

▶▶ 2 Scotch pancakes (see page 153) filled with 1 sliced banana and a tablespoon of raisins or sultanas, and two tablespoons of plain low-fat yoghurt or plain low-fat fromage frais.

▶▶ Small glass of milk.

Chicken/ham sandwich

This is a great one if you are short of time as you can make the sandwich the night before, wrap it in cling film, and put it in the fridge until breakfast time.

▶▶ A banana.

▶▶ Chicken or lean ham sandwich (use wholemeal bread and buy a slice of 'real' ham from a joint not processed or 'reformed' ham).

▶▶ Small glass of milk.

Egg and soldiers

▶▶ An apple cut into wedges.

▶▶ Boiled egg and wholemeal toast 'soldiers' for dipping (no butter or spread).

▶▶ Small glass of milk.

Sardines on toast

▶▶ A banana.

▶▶ ½ can sardines in tomato sauce, grilled on wholemeal toast.

▶▶ Small glass of milk.

Open sandwich

▶▶ Fruit of your choice.

▶▶ Open sandwich made with one thick slice of wholemeal bread topped with low-fat cream cheese, slices of banana, and a drizzle of runny honey. Eat with a knife and fork.

▶▶ Small glass of milk.

Breakfast bagel

▶▶ A banana.

▶▶ Wholegrain bagel or slice of thick wholemeal toast topped with 'healthy' peanut butter, low-fat cream cheese or low-sugar jam.

▶▶ Small glass of milk.

English muffin

▶▶ An apple cut into wedges.

▶▶ Half a wholemeal English muffin toasted and topped with a tablespoon of natural yogurt, fresh berries and a drizzle of honey.

▶▶ Small glass of milk.

Grilled tomato and mushrooms

▶▶ A banana.

▶▶ Grilled tomato and mushroom on a toasted wholemeal English muffin.

▶▶ Small glass of milk.

Breakfast sundae

▶▶ A breakfast sundae (made the night before). Layer fresh or tinned fruit in juice and a small fromage frais or yoghurt in a glass and put in the fridge. In the morning top with 1–2 tablespoons of no-sugar muesli or low-sugar cereal.

▶▶ A small glass of milk.

Cheese omelette

▶▶ A banana.

▶▶ A cheese omelette and grilled tomato.

▶▶ A small glass of milk.

choosing a cereal

There's a bewildering array of breakfast cereals out there, ranging from the ultra-healthy to the absolutely dire.

Top cereals for kids:

▶▶ Porridge – go for porridge oats rather than 'instant' oats. Coarse oats provide slower-release energy, and the instant versions are often high in sugar.

▶▶ Muesli – go for one with no added sugar or salt. Beware of 'crunchy' oat cereals that look a bit like muesli. Those little clusters are stuck together with sugars.

▶▶ Shredded wheat cereals (no added sugar, and low salt). Children generally prefer the bite-sized versions.

▶▶ Weetabix-type biscuits – the 'plain' ones are best, check the sugar content in the bite-sized versions with added raisins etc.

Plus point:

▶▶ Fortification – many cereals are fortified with vitamins and minerals, such as the B vitamins, and iron. This can give an important boost to children's nutrient intake – fortified breakfast cereals contribute an average of 29% of boys' iron intake, and 23% of girls' iron. But you shouldn't buy a highly sweetened, ultra-refined cereal just because it's had vitamins added to it. It's far better to buy something that's ultra-healthy in the first place, such as porridge or no-sugar muesli.

Watchpoint:

▶▶ Wholegrain is good, but many wholegrain cereals are still horribly high in sugar.

WEEK 4 - LUNCH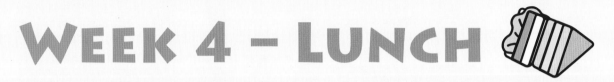

A child's lunch should contain at least a third of their requirements for protein, 'healthy' fats, carbohydrates, vitamins and minerals, and no more than a third of their recommended daily maximum for total fat, saturated fat, salt and added sugar.

A tall order? Not really, if you give your child a healthy home-prepared meal.

Sadly, many children's lunches are far from healthy.

schoolday lunches

In the past, school dinners in the UK had a dreadful reputation – nutritionally poor, and chips with everything! Now that there are new, tougher laws governing school dinners, to prevent the serving and selling of 'junk foods' in schools, and to ensure that there are plenty of fruits, vegetables, semi-skimmed milk, wholemeal products, water and other products available, you might think that a school meal is the healthiest option for your child.

But things are never that simple! Even if a school provides the healthiest meals in the world, there's no guarantee that the children will eat them! It's impossible to force a child to choose a balanced meal from the school cafeteria – even if all the 'right' options are available.

If your child has school meals, encourage them to make the best choices so that they do get a balanced meal. Most schools will provide parents with a lunch menu, so that you can look at it with your child and help them to choose a sustaining and balanced lunch.

Packed lunches have the potential to be extremely healthy – after all, you control what goes into them. But all too often they are nutritionally dire – just as bad as the 'old style' school dinners. A survey of packed lunches by the Food Standards Agency found that they contained too much saturated fat, sugar, and especially salt. Sixty-nine per cent of lunchboxes contained a packet of crisps and 58% included a chocolate bar or biscuits.

And many of the items sold in supermarkets and shops as good for packed lunches are higher in fat, salt and sugar than is healthy for a child.

There's nothing wrong with crisps or chocolate occasionally – but it's not good for children to have them every day in their packed lunches. And special 'lunchbox food' from the supermarket can be a real time saver. But it's so much healthier (not to mention cheaper) to make your own versions of these gimmicky products.

So, for the purpose of this book, our 6-Week Junk-Free Plan explains how to devise healthy packed lunches *with* your child. Note: 'with', not 'for' your child. This is an opportunity to really let them get involved in choosing what goes into their meal (but within your healthy guidelines). This way they're more likely to enjoy and eat everything in their lunchbox.

If your child has school lunches, we'll also tell you how to help them make the best 'junk-free' choices.

the junk-free pick-&-mix lunchbox plan

Before each school week, sit down with your child and plan the week's packed lunches.

Pick one item from each of the lists. No fizzy drinks!! No junk food!

In other words, one of each of these:

▶▶ **1 main bit**

▶▶ **1 fruit & veg**

▶▶ **1 calcium bone builder**

▶▶ **1 drink**

▶▶ **1 treat**

The main bit

Sandwiches can become boring, so ring the changes by using different kinds of breads. Simply choose one of these fillings and use it to make a sandwich or fill a fajita wrap or chapatti, a pitta bread pocket, a bread roll, a bagel or low-salt wholewheat crackers. Choose wholemeal so long as it doesn't fill your child up too much. If they won't eat wholemeal bread use one of the new high fibre white breads or try one of the speciality breads like walnut, multi grain, or sun-dried tomato. Add as much lettuce and sliced tomato and cucumber to any of these as you like.

If you want to try out an unfamiliar filling on your child, and are worried that they won't like it and will go hungry at lunchtime, why not serve a half size portion as an after school snack or try out a couple for weekend garden picnic lunch.

Filling Ideas

▶▶ Sliced poached chicken breast, low-fat mayonnaise and finely chopped salad vegetables

▶▶ Tinned salmon (drain, and remove the skin), chopped cucumber and low-fat mayonnaise or salad cream

▶▶ Chopped hardboiled egg, cress and low-fat mayonnaise or salad cream

▶▶ Tinned tuna with finely chopped cucumber, and lettuce

▶▶ Peanut butter (not too much!) and sliced or mashed banana

▶▶ Sliced roast turkey and low-fat coleslaw

▶▶ Low-fat grated cheese with apple slices and lettuce

▶▶ Drained low-fat cottage cheese, grated carrot and grated apple

▶▶ Low-fat cream cheese, tomato, cucumber and lettuce

▶▶ Hardboiled egg slices with cress and a teaspoon of low-fat salad cream

▶▶ Chopped roast chicken and 1 tablespoon of low-fat coleslaw

▶▶ Lettuce, tomato and low-fat coleslaw, topped with two small slices of lean ham

▶▶ Peanut butter with sliced cucumber

▶▶ Low-fat cream cheese and banana slices

▶▶ Sliced vegetarian sausage with pickle and lettuce

Alternatives to Sandwiches

As an alternative to a sandwich sometimes, older children may like a pasta or rice salad with some cooked chicken, tinned salmon or tuna. Or how about a slice of homemade quiche or some homemade soup and a roll?

The fruit or veg

▶▶ A small bunch of grapes

▶▶ A Satsuma, Mandarin or Clementine

▶▶ An orange

▶▶ A banana

▶▶ A pear

▶▶ A nectarine/peach

▶▶ A small carton or tin of fruit in juice (remember to pack a spoon)

▶▶ A pot of washed berries

▶▶ A kiwifruit (cut it in half, then put back together and wrap in cling film. Give your child a teaspoon to scoop the flesh out)

▶▶ A selection of veggie sticks – celery, carrot, pepper, cucumber, small florets of cauliflower or broccoli. (You can also include a yoghurt based dip or a little cottage cheese in a small container for dipping)

▶▶ 5 cherry tomatoes

▶▶ 2 small tomatoes, cut into wedges

The calcium bone builder

Remember that many yoghurts targeted at children are high in sugar, colouring and other additives, so go for those that are as low in sugar and as 'natural' as possible. Plain natural yoghurt is best of all – give your child a little pot of fruit purée, honey or chopped dried fruit to add to it if they don't like 'plain' yoghurt.

▶▶ A small carton of yoghurt

▶▶ A small bottle of drinking yoghurt

▶▶ Small carton of fromage frais

▶▶ 3 tablespoons of cottage cheese with pineapple (in a small plastic tub)

You can, if you like, leave out the calcium bone builder if the sandwich filling chosen contains cheese. But leave it in if you think your child's meal won't be sustaining enough otherwise.

The treats

▶▶ A finger of fruity bar (see page 157)

▶▶ A mini hot cross bun or currant bun

▶▶ 1 tablespoon sultanas or raisins

▶▶ 4 unsulphured dried apricots or dried mango slices

▶▶ A child-sized handful of mixed nuts and seeds

▶▶ Low-sugar flapjack (see page 158)

▶▶ An oatcake or digestive biscuit

▶▶ A Garibaldi biscuit or fig roll

▶▶ A small low-sugar muffin (see page 156)

▶▶ A fruit scone

▶▶ A small plastic tub filled with plain popcorn

▶▶ A small slice of malt loaf or fruit bread

Don't stress yourself if your child wants to have the same sandwich or treat in their lunchbox EVERY single day. Just make sure that they get plenty of variety elsewhere in their lunch, and in their other meals. The chances are, it won't be too long before they get fed up with eggy wrap or whatever it was, and ask for something different.

LUNCHBOX SAFETY

Use an insulated lunchbox, and a small ice pack to keep food cold. It's a good idea to prepare part or all of the packed lunch the evening before and store the food and drinks in the fridge. They'll be well chilled when you put them into the lunchbox, with the icepack.

Wash and dry lunchboxes each evening.

Once a week treats

Add one of these special treats to the lunchbox each week (instead of an item from the treats list, not as well as!):

▶▶ A small packet of pretzels

▶▶ A small packet of low-fat, low-salt crisps

▶▶ A tablespoon of yoghurt-covered raisins – once a week only

▶▶ A snack-sized chocolate bar

▶▶ A chocolate-coated biscuit

▶▶ A small 'shop-bought' cake

▶▶ A small gingerbread person (check that it doesn't contain hydrogenated fats)

The drink

▶▶ Pure fruit juice, diluted ½ juice, ½ water

▶▶ A bottle of plain water (not flavoured or sweetened)

(Your child should also always drink at least a glass of water at lunchtime.)

what to do if your child has school lunches

Choosing a healthy lunch at school

If you get a copy of the school meals menu from your child's school you will be able to help them to plan some healthy lunches that they're happy to eat (at least most of the time) from the wide range of items on offer. Explain to them which are the healthy options and why.

Try to persuade them to choose:

▶▶ A pasta dish with a tomato or vegetable sauce

▶▶ A jacket potato filled with baked beans, tuna, coleslaw, or cottage cheese

▶▶ A vegetable bake

▶▶ Stews and casseroles

▶▶ Non-fried chicken or fish dishes

▶▶ Vegetable or chicken soups

▶▶ Salads with meat, cheese or fish (but without oily dressings)

And to AVOID, except on rare occasions, anything on the following list. (Perhaps you could negotiate what constitutes 'rare' – say once a fortnight? And then only one item.)

▶▶ Chips

▶▶ Roast potatoes

▶▶ Fried fish

▶▶ Burgers

▶▶ Chicken nuggets

▶▶ Sausages

▶▶ Creamy pasta dishes

For dessert, steer them towards fruit or a yoghurt instead of cakes, cookies, sponge puddings and pies.

As far as drinks are concerned ask them to choose water, diluted fruit juice or milk.

There's no guarantee that you'll actually persuade them to eat what you think is best when they get into the dining room, but if they develop a taste for fresh, healthy food at home they're more likely, over time, to prefer healthier choices.

weekend and school holiday lunches

During the weekends and school holidays you'll probably want something quick and easy at lunchtime. But that's no reason to let the junk creep in!

Here are some ideas for quick and healthy lunches. You'll find the recipes for the meals marked with a 📖 at the end of this book. If your family likes to have their main meal at lunchtime on Sunday then feel free to swap dinner and lunch on that day.

▶▶ A bowl of quick Chunky Homemade Chunky Vegetable and Pasta Soup with a warmed crusty roll 📖

▶▶ A cheese, mushroom or ham omelette with grilled tomatoes and peas and potato wedges 📖

▶▶ Quick Crusty Pizza with a large green salad 📖

▶▶ Potato wedges with grilled Quorn sausage, baked beans and grilled tomato 📖

▶▶ A small baked jacket potato filled with a little tuna and sweetcorn, low-fat coleslaw, grated carrot and raisins, chopped cooked chicken with sweetcorn and a little low-fat mayo, low-sugar, low-salt baked beans. Serve with a salad

▶▶ A mixed salad of sliced new potatoes, lettuce, cucumber, tomato topped with a little low-fat dressing and some strips of cooked chicken or tinned salmon. Serve with crusty bread or boiled new potatoes

▶▶ Sweet sesame chicken strips with brown rice and salad 📖

▶▶ Stuffed ham cones with new potatoes and salad. Take a slice of ham, roll it into a cone shape and fill with a mixture of sweetcorn and peas combined with a little low-fat mayonnaise.

▶▶ Chicken Dippers with Tomato Dip and Peas and Sweetcorn Mash 📖

▶▶ Baked beans and grilled tomatoes on toast

▶▶ Homemade beef, chicken, turkey or bean burger with a toasted wholemeal burger bun and salad 📖

▶▶ Tinned sardines on wholemeal toast with low-fat coleslaw

▶▶ Homemade Potato Wedgie Bowl 📖

▶▶ Baked potato with topping and salad 📖

▶▶ Pronto Pasta and Sauce 📖

Offer a piece of fruit or a small glass of milk for dessert.

WEEK 5 – DINNER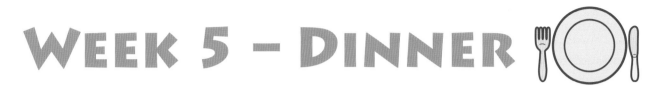

making mealtimes happy times

Nowadays, our modern lifestyles mean that the traditional family sit-down dinner seems to be becoming a thing of the past. Parents may not arrive back from work until relatively late in the evening, and when we do get home, cooking can be the last thing we want to do. In situations like this, getting the children's meal out of the way as quickly as possible, and then eating a microwave ready meal from a tray on your lap in front of the TV, can seem very tempting!

Some parents give their children a 'quick kid's meal' of something like fish fingers or pizza and chips, pretty soon after they get home from school, and then cook their own dinner later, often after the children have gone to bed. This may seem the easier option, but it's far from ideal.

For a start, it teaches children that there's 'kid food' and there's 'grown-up food'. Whether they think kid food is more 'fun' than adult food, or feel short-changed because they think the meal you're having yourselves later is somehow 'better', this isn't a healthy attitude for them.

If you don't eat with your children regularly, you also lose the opportunity to be their healthy-eating role models. You can't over-emphasise the influence of parents' eating habits on their children's food choices – both now and in the future. By demonstrating what you want them to do, you're making it so much easier for them to learn important lessons for the future.

Also, children often need encouragement to try new foods. Remember the scenes in *Jamie Oliver's School*

OUT AND ABOUT

If you're away from home at lunchtime, it's all too tempting to stop at a fast food restaurant for something to eat. And occasionally – once a month or so – that's OK. But fast food isn't good as a regular choice and can also be expensive. If you know you're going to be out and about at lunchtime, take packed lunches for the whole family. If you all abide by the 'lunchbox rules', choosing from the lists above, your children will know they're worth following! We'll also give you more advice on eating 'on the hoof' in Part 3.

Dinners TV programmes, where little 'junk-food addicts' initially turned up their noses at Jamie's healthy creations, but were gradually cajoled into eating and enjoying them? It took time, and effort. You can't expect a child to try something new if you just dump the plate in front of them and then leave. If you're sitting with them, however, and taking an interest in what they're doing, you can coax them, and praise them when they try a little bit – and you're much more likely to be successful.

Eating together as a family is a really valuable experience, so it's worth making the effort to eat together at least once a day, whether it's breakfast, lunch or dinner. Eating together isn't only enjoyable, it also helps children to learn social skills such as the importance of sharing, politeness and consideration for others.

Try to avoid leaving a child to eat on their own, as it can be a very lonely experience, and will often mean that the child eats only a little of their meal so that they can move on to doing something they think is more interesting. If something prevents you from having your 'proper' meal at the same time as your child, try to sit with them when they are eating. At least have a cup of tea and a piece of fruit (preferably cut into slices on a plate so that it looks like a meal).

But don't watch over the child like a hawk – imagine how intimidated you would feel!

Make mealtimes a relaxed 'grumble free zone'. Keep criticisms and complaints for later and ask your child to do the same.

Many families have the television on during mealtimes, or allow the children to eat their meals in front of the TV. But this really is a big distraction – your child should be concentrating on their meal, not the screen, so turn it off!

Families who have a sit-down dinner together tend to eat healthier dinners than those who eat separately. It makes sense – if you have to prepare one meal for yourself, another for your partner who might get home at a different time, and

yet another for the children, you're more likely to grab convenience foods like frozen pizzas and ready meals.

Many people think that a home-cooked meal for all the family is really time consuming and just too much hassle, particularly after a hard day's work. Or that it won't 'keep' if one person can't eat with the rest.

But this needn't be the case – food you prepare yourself can be just as convenient as 'convenience food' – if you choose something simple and plan ahead.

the junk-free dinner plan

Using the suggested weekly menu plan below, choose an appropriate recipe from the menu choices to match the day. You'll find all these simple recipes at the end of the book.

Weekly menu
▶▶ **SUNDAY is Chicken Day**
▶▶ **MONDAY is Fish Day**
▶▶ **TUESDAY is Beans Day**
▶▶ **WEDNESDAY is You Choose Day**
▶▶ **THURSDAY is Chicken Day or Vegetarian Day**
▶▶ **FRIDAY is Fish Day**
▶▶ **SATURDAY is You Choose Day**

'You Choose Day' means you can have any recipe you like from the meal plan. Perhaps you could let the children choose the dinner dish.

When the weather is fine, how about eating outside? You'll be amazed at what it does for the appetite. You don't have to make anything special or fire up the barbecue, just carry your plates outside and enjoy the food and the sunshine.

Dinner menu choices

Chicken Day

▶▶ Hot Baked Chicken with Mashed Potato and Fresh Boiled Vegetables

▶▶ Speedy Chicken and Vegetable Stir-fry with Brown Rice or Noodles

▶▶ Muffin Chicken Pizza with Salad

▶▶ Baked Chicken Breast with Sweetcorn Mash and Fresh Boiled Vegetables

▶▶ Spanish Chicken with Pasta and Green Salad

▶▶ Turkey Burger with Chunky Oven Chips and Green Salad

Fish Day

▶▶ Pan-cooked Cod or Haddock Fillet with Homemade Chunky Chips and Vegetables

▶▶ Pan-fried Fresh Salmon with Boiled New Potatoes and Vegetables

▶▶ Homemade Fish Fingers with Chunky Chips, Peas and Grilled Tomatoes

▶▶ Baked Cod with Breadcrumb Topping, Mashed Potatoes and a Selection of Vegetables or Green Salad

▶▶ Speedy Tuna or Salmon and Tomato Pasta with Salad

▶▶ Prawn and Vegetable Stir-fry with Rice or Noodles

Beans Day

▶▶ Spicy Lentil Casserole with Brown Rice or Boiled New Potatoes and Fresh Vegetables or Salad

▶▶ Chickpea and Vegetable Chilli with Brown Rice and a Green Salad or Fresh Boiled Vegetables

▶▶ Cowboy Sausage and Beans with Mashed (or Jacket) Potato and Broccoli

▶▶ Oven-Baked Bean Burgers with a Wholemeal Bap and Salad

▶▶ Spicy Bean Fajita Wraps with a Green Salad

▶▶ Beany Braise with Green Vegetables and Crusty Bread

Vegetarian Day

▶▶ Cowboy Sausage and Beans with Mashed (or Jacket) Potato and Broccoli

▶▶ Veggie Frittata with a Green Salad and Wholemeal Bap

▶▶ Egg and Mushroom Pan-fry with a Salad and Warmed Wholemeal Bap

▶▶ Broccoli, Cauliflower and Sweetcorn Cheese, with Boiled New Potatoes and Grilled Tomatoes

▶▶ Vegetarian Sausage Topper with Baked Beans, Grilled Tomatoes, Jacket Potato and Salad and Low-fat Coleslaw

▶▶ Mild Egg and Vegetable Curry with Rice

▶▶ Pepper and Tomato Pasta with Salad or Broccoli and Crusty Bread

Sweet endings

Desserts are always welcome after a main meal, and they can be simple and quick – some don't need any preparation at all. More complex desserts can be kept for special occasions.

On most days a piece of fruit, a yoghurt, a fromage frais, or a combination of these will be perfect. But you may need the hard sell to convince children that fruit is 'pudding'. This is a time when a couple of minutes spent making it look attractive can pay dividends. Chunks of fruit on wooden skewers or a platter of fruits in fan shapes always look more appealing than simply asking a child to grab something from the fruit bowl. Or how about cutting an apple into horizontal slices and then reconstructing it, or standing strawberries or raspberries on a slice of melon so they look like 'sailors' on a boat.

Here are some ideas for simple desserts and some special occasion desserts:

▶▶ A bowl of tinned fruit (canned in juice not syrup) with yoghurt or fromage frais

▶▶ Some slices of fresh pineapple, grilled and served with yoghurt or fromage frais

▶▶ A bowl of mixed seasonal fruit soaked in a little orange juice and topped with yoghurt, a teaspoon of chopped nuts and a drizzle of honey or maple syrup

▶▶ Puréed mango spooned over natural yoghurt

▶▶ A slice of melon with a small carton of fromage frais

▶▶ A small carton of low-fat rice pudding with some fresh berry fruits or nectarine wedges

▶▶ A couple of squares of good quality chocolate

Special Desserts

(You'll find the recipes at the back of the book)

▶▶ Plum and Almond Crumble

▶▶ Baked Bananas

▶▶ Strawberry Meringue Delight

▶▶ Scotch Pancake Stack with Berry Fruits and Quark

▶▶ Orangey Pears with Fromage Frais

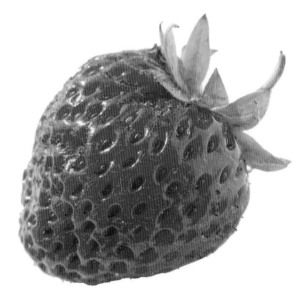

WEEK 6 – SNACKS: SORTED!

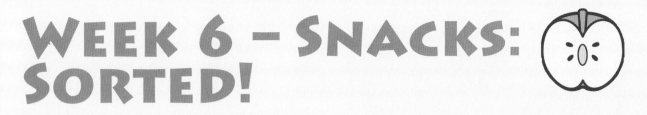

You (and your child) will be relieved to learn that snacks aren't banned when you de-junk your child's diet. On the contrary – snacks don't have to be nutritional disasters, and they're an essential part of the 6-Week Junk-Free Plan, and beyond.

You simply have to remember that there are healthy snacks and less healthy snacks. We're going to replace most of the less healthy snacks with tasty, nutritious ones – so there's still room for the occasional chocolate bar.

Why do children need healthy snacks?

▶▶ Children have small stomachs – they can't eat enough at a sitting to keep them going until the next meal.

▶▶ Snacks make it easier for children to get enough of all the nutrients they need – this is particularly important if your child has a small appetite and can't eat a lot at mealtimes.

▶▶ Snacks help maintain stable blood sugar levels, by allowing children to 're-fuel' regularly. This stops children from getting hungry and cranky.

▶▶ If a child eats a healthy snack, they're less likely to be tempted by one that's packed with sugar, fat or salt, than if they're hungry.

▶▶ Snacks are an excellent opportunity to slip a fruit or vegetable portion into your child's diet.

▶▶ Snacks that include a drink help children to stay hydrated.

▶▶ Snacking is part of most children's lives – they'd feel deprived if snacks were banned.

Saying that snacks are allowed is not the same as saying children can graze whenever they like. Like meals, snacks should have a set time – obviously this can be flexible within reason, but snacks aren't an 'anytime thing'. Children need to learn when 'snack time' is – they shouldn't think of them as random handouts. Nor should they be able to ask for a snack whenever they want.

Snacks should be mini-meals, approximately midway between their main meals.

▶▶ Long enough after the meal before, so that your child knows they'll have to wait a while if they don't eat what's on their plate.

▶▶ Long enough before the next meal, so as not to spoil the child's appetite.

When snack time arrives, make sure you have the snack ready and prepared. If you're caught on the hop, your child may have decided what they want, and it may not be the healthy option you had in mind. If the snack is ready and waiting, there's less opportunity for your child to launch into an argument.

Mid-morning and as soon as they get home from school are particularly good times for snacks, but you'll know when fits in best with your lifestyle.

WORKING TOGETHER

Sit down with your child at the beginning of the school term and have a meeting about what they're going to have for snacks. They'll appreciate being treated like an adult.

Have a brainstorming session together, coming up with a selection of nutritious snacks, and agree to throw in a very occasional snack-sized chocolate bar or packet of low-fat crisps. If a child knows they can have crisps and chocolate sometimes, they're more likely to be happy with healthier snacks the rest of the time.

Don't be surprised if your child comes up with some strange snack suggestions – to many children, the ultimate snack is a weird and wonderful combination of two or more of their favourite foods. Sweet and savoury together seem to be particularly popular.

- If they want peanut butter and apple, why not? Just core an apple, cut it into horizontal slices, spread the slices with a healthy low-sugar low-salt peanut butter, then put the apple back together again. Wrap in foil or cling film.
- How about celery and raisins? Fill the 'hollow' of the celery stick with raisins, then wrap in cling film or foil.
- The 'peanut butter and jelly sandwich' is a famous American taste sensation. Use wholemeal bread and a 'healthy' peanut butter – you won't need butter or spread. The 'jelly' is jam, so use a low-sugar high-fruit version.

Sweet or savoury – get to know your child's 'snack personality'

One child may adore chocolate bars, another may be more of a crisp fan. And your child may hanker for different snacks at different times. For example, they may like something savoury during morning break, especially if their friends are eating crisps, but might fancy something sweet when they come home from school.

You need to learn what kind of snacker your child is, because you'll have more success in persuading them to eat healthy snacks, if the snacks you give them fit in with their idea of what they wanted.

If, for example, you try to replace a chocolate bar snack with celery sticks and a savoury dip, you'll probably run up against opposition. But a couple of sweet but sustaining fig rolls are more likely to be an acceptable swap. And if your child always has a savoury snack attack at a certain time of day – say, a packet of crisps after school – try offering them a snack such as breadsticks or oatcakes and low-fat cream cheese, rather than a sweet fruit snack, or a healthy homemade bake.

What makes a good children's snack?

▶▶ It should be a food the child enjoys
▶▶ It should be sustaining, to keep the child going until the next meal
▶▶ It should be 'nutrient dense' – as much nutrition as possible in a small package
▶▶ It should be low in fat, salt and sugar
▶▶ It should be easy-to-eat 'finger food'
▶▶ It should be portable in the case of snacks for taking to school

▶▶ It should ideally contain two out of the following three:
Fruit/vegetables
Protein – nuts, cheese, milk, yoghurt
Starchy carbohydrate

the junk-free snack plan
Morning snacks

On school days, a healthy snack for eating during morning break will top up your child's energy levels until lunchtime. Many schools encourage, and even sell, snacks for this time, but all too often they're of the chocolate and crisps variety.

Encouragingly, more and more schools are selling fruit at break time or, even better, have a free fruit scheme. But be ready for the fact that many of your child's friends will be eating sugary chocolate bars, sweets and crisps – not what you want to encourage. Your snacks need to compete with the junk snacks – it's a tough brief – but not impossible.

A school snack also needs to be simple to eat and well packed – your child won't eat it if it's turned to mush or crumbs in their school bag!

And of course, your child will still need a morning snack on non-school days.

Afternoon snacks

As the afternoon snack will often be eaten when your child gets home from school, this is an excellent opportunity to get healthy food inside your child, and to introduce new foods, when they will probably be hungry and willing to try something they might otherwise turn up their noses at.

If you're struggling to get a particular food group into your child's diet – they're reluctant to eat dairy, fruit or vegetables, for example – this is the time to slip it in.

Working the plan

Just choose a morning snack and an afternoon snack for each day.

On weekdays, it's best to have this snack straight after school, but at weekends and non-school days, try to have it as close to mid-way between lunch and supper as possible. If you need to take your child to a class or activity straight after school, take the snack with you.

As you did with breakfasts, lunches and suppers, encourage your child to choose as wide a selection as possible, to ensure the maximum possible variety of foods and nutrients.

We've also included some 'occasional snacks' in our list – your child can have one of those every week. These are the ones that in an ideal world wouldn't be there – chocolate bars, crisps and the like. But if you ban this kind of snack completely, your child will probably dig their little heels in and refuse to co-operate. Children will be children, and if allowing them a 'naughty' snack every now and then means they'll eat healthier snacks the rest of the time, it's a price worth paying. And if it stops them from looking too 'different' from other children who don't eat so healthily, they'll be more likely to enjoy their new 'Snacking Plan'. But don't make the mistake of actually calling these snacks 'naughty', or 'treats' – you don't want your child to think there's something special about them.

Snacks need to be quick to prepare and simple for the child to eat, particularly if they're on the move. If you have time some can be prepared in advance, so that all you have to do is take them out of the fridge.

Try to sit down with your child when they have their afternoon snack. It will give you a few minutes' breather and it's a good time for them to tell you about their day and any little worries they may have. Far better to deal with them now than at bedtime!

The snacks

Keep snacks small, you don't want to dampen down your child's appetite but you do need to provide energy and stave off hunger pangs.

Sweet snacks

▶▶ Slices of apple, banana, and a few grapes with a couple of tablespoons of fromage frais.

▶▶ A kiwifruit or a slice of pineapple with fromage frais.

▶▶ A fruit kebab – cold or lightly grilled with yoghurt or fromage frais.

▶▶ A low-fat fromage frais or fruit yoghurt.

▶▶ Wholemeal toast fingers with low-fat cottage cheese and pineapple.

▶▶ 2 oatcakes with cottage cheese and a few sultanas and seeds sprinkled over.

▶▶ A toasted English muffin with fruit spread or low-sugar jam.

▶▶ 2 digestive biscuits sandwiched together with a little low-fat cream cheese.

▶▶ A slice of malt loaf.

▶▶ A toasted currant bun spread with low-sugar jam.

▶▶ A homemade Fruity bar, Muesli square or Oat jack finger (see page 157).

▶▶ A handful of granola (see page 159).

▶▶ A warmed scotch pancake (see page 153) topped with a handful of berries and a tablespoon of low-fat yoghurt or fromage frais.

▶▶ A handful of dried fruit and seeds sprinkled over a small bowl of natural yoghurt. Drizzle a little honey over.

▶▶ A small homemade Fast fruity muffin (see page 156).

Savoury snacks

▶▶ Veggie sticks – try carrot, celery, cucumber and pepper – with a yoghurt-based dip or low-fat hummus.

▶▶ Sticks of celery filled with low-fat cream cheese.

▶▶ A small bowl of vegetable soup and a slice of wholemeal toast.

▶▶ A hardboiled egg and a slice of wholemeal bread spread with low-fat spread.

▶▶ A small slice of cooked chicken or lean ham with a small wholemeal roll spread with low-fat spread.

▶▶ 2 wholemeal crackers spread with low-fat soft cheese and a few slices of apple.

▶▶ Wholemeal toast fingers spread with peanut butter or low-fat soft cheese.

▶▶ Half a small bagel topped with egg and cress, or low-fat cream cheese.

▶▶ A small bowl of plain popcorn with a little low-fat cheese finely grated over it.

Occasional snacks

If 'occasional snacks' appear as part of your normal snack repertoire your child shouldn't feel they're any different from other children or being deprived of what they believe are the good things in life. The lure of less healthy snacks will hopefully be reduced. They'll see that the things they 'really like' have not been banned, so they'll be less likely to constantly want them.

You can have one of these occasional treats in each week's plan:

▶▶ A small bowl of low-fat crisps (look for ones which are cooked (preferably oven baked) in vegetable oil, not hydrogenated vegetable oil, and also low in salt). Plus a piece of fresh fruit.

▶▶ A small bowl of pretzels or tortilla chips with a piece of fresh fruit.

▶▶ A small chocolate biscuit bar.

▶▶ A snack-sized chocolate bar.

▶▶ 2 biscuits or cookies – choose those with the healthiest ingredients, or make them yourself.

▶▶ A scoop of good quality ice cream. Look for one with 'real' ingredients like cream, milk and sugar, rather than a huge list full of chemicals!

▶▶ A small iced fairy cake (preferably homemade, to cut out the trans fats and other nasty additives).

If you serve items like crisps and pretzels in small bowls, they won't realise if you don't give them the whole packet in one go.

ADAPTING THE SIX-WEEK PLAN

The 6-Week Junk-Free Plan is designed for healthy primary school-aged children (7–11), who don't need to lose any weight. But it can easily be adapted if your child doesn't fit into that category.

Use the plan as a guide, but tweak the portions sizes according to your child's needs, and substitute alternative meals if they're more appropriate. The recipes in the plan have symbols showing you whether they're good sources of particular nutrients, to make this easy for you. For example, look out for the symbol if you're after a meal that's a good source of iron.

children who need to lose weight

Hardly a day goes by when childhood obesity isn't in the news. On the whole, modern children don't have any problems in growing – today's children are taller, on average, than previous generations. The problem is, a lot of them are also growing 'outwards'.

Believe it or not, 28% of children aged 2–10 are overweight, and 14 % are obese (extremely overweight), and the figures are rising. It's no fun being an overweight child. Larger children are more likely to be bullied at school, and their confidence suffers. Sometimes this can lead to depression.

Children of a healthy weight, on the other hand, are more likely to:

▸▸ Enjoy sports and physical activity.

▸▸ Have plenty of confidence, in everyday life and in lessons.

▸▸ Have good self esteem, and find it easier to make friends.

Weighing too much makes it harder for children to fulfil their potential – they're more likely to struggle with lessons, hate sports because they find them harder and more tiring, find it harder to make friends and suffer more from poor self esteem.

The benefits of maintaining the correct weight aren't just emotional and academic – it's positively good for your child's health.

▸▸ Healthy weight children are more likely to maintain their weight in adulthood.

▸▸ Healthy weight children have a decreased risk of heart disease, stroke and type 2 diabetes later in life. Being overweight is one of the main causes of high blood pressure, increased cholesterol levels and poor blood sugar control – all of which are risk factors for these serious illnesses.

▸▸ Healthy weight children have a lower risk of certain cancers later in life. Being overweight over a period of many years increases the risk.

Changing your family's diet for the better, to help an overweight child to lose weight, can really have a dramatic – and wonderful – effect. And as they lose the troublesome pounds, they'll also find that they have more energy, and simply 'feel' better.

losing weight and the 6-week junk-free plan

Here's the good news. If you or your child are carrying too many pounds because you were previously eating badly, all you need to do is eat healthily, become more active and increase the amount of exercise you all do. Then you'll lose the excess weight – gradually, safely, and sustainably.

Your child doesn't need to 'go on a diet'.

Luckily, our healthy diet plan doesn't mean deprivation or hunger – you and your child will probably find you're eating more food than before. Healthy foods are generally lower in calories than 'junk food', so by switching to healthier options you can eat more and weigh less, which can't be bad!

Crash diets are a bad idea – for anyone, but most especially for children. So you won't see any of that in this book!

A far better solution to prevent your child from becoming overweight in the first place, or to help an overweight child to lose weight, is for the whole family to embark on a healthy diet that's junk-free as far as possible – and this book shows you how. Any excess weight was probably gained because a child ate too many calories while not burning enough energy.

This means that if they stick to the recommended calorie intake, while increasing their activity levels (you can learn more about this in Part 3), it should prevent any further weight gain and lead to a slow and gradual weight loss. This is far safer and more sustainable than a strict weight loss diet.

You need to concentrate on the positive, not the negative. Say that you're changing some of the things you all eat because you want to be healthier and feel better, not that you're cutting out treats to lose weight.

DON'T SAY:
'You can't have chips and burgers because they're bad for you.'
DO SAY:
'We're going to eat more fruit and vegetables because they're good for us.'

DON'T SAY:
'We're not going to have takeaways because they're full of fat.'
DO SAY:
'We're going to do more cooking at home because it's fun and we can have more choice about what we eat.'

how to adapt the 6-week junk-free plan if your child needs to lose weight

If your child has stubborn pounds that won't seem to shift, even despite their best healthy-eating and exercise efforts, try these tips:

▶▶ Slightly increasing the fibre in their diet – replacing any refined 'white' foods with unprocessed, wholemeal or 'brown' versions. This should help them feel sustained between meals.

▶▶ Slightly decrease the size of portions for carbohydrate foods, such as potatoes, pasta, rice and bread. Please note that we're in no way recommending a 'low-carb' diet! It's vital for children to eat enough carbohydrates. Over time, a very small reduction of approximately 10–15% in their carbohydrate intake should help with weight loss. These carbohydrates can be replaced once the child's weight has stabilised at a healthy level.

▶▶ Hold off the 'Occasional Snacks' in the plan – just for now.

▶▶ Make sure they have plenty of fruit and vegetables to fill them up and for snacks – they're low in calories, and high in vitamins, minerals and fibre. Exceptions, which should be limited to once a day because they're higher in calories, are bananas, parsnips, sweetcorn, sweet potatoes and potatoes.

▶▶ Switch from semi-skimmed to skimmed milk, and always choose the lowest fat version of foods such as dairy products.

▶▶ Make sure your child is drinking enough water – sometimes children think they're hungry when they're really just thirsty.

And remember, you also need to increase their activity levels, so that they burn up more energy. Turn to Part 4 for our child-friendly exercise advice.

Stay positive and encouraging – you can do it!

adapting the plan for younger children

Slightly younger children (say, aged 4–6) can also benefit from cutting down on less healthy food, using a modified version of the 6-Week Junk Free Plan.

Younger children have slightly different nutritional needs, and you can see from the table below that they require smaller portions.

These are the estimated average calorie requirements for younger children:

Age (years)	Calories (boys)	Calories (girls)
4–6	1,715	1,545
7–10	1,970	1,740

It's also important to know that the recommended maximum amount of salt is set lower for younger children.

4–6-year olds	Maximum 3g salt (1.2g sodium)
7–10-year-olds	Maximum 5g salt (2g sodium)

You'll also need to use different tactics to persuade younger children to eat healthily – this is the age group where presentation comes into its own. Try food made into 'faces', 'flowers' or 'trains' on the plate, sandwiches cut into funny shapes, and 'finger food' – things like veggie sticks and bread sticks with a healthy dip.

And here's a big plus point for parents of little ones – you have more control over younger children's diets, giving you the opportunity to help them to form healthy food preferences that will last them for life.

adapting the plan for older children

You can also adapt the 6-Week Junk Free Plan for slightly older children (say, 11–14 years old).

Like younger children, teenagers are growing rapidly, and they need foods dense in nutrients.

Once again, their calorie requirements have increased, so they can have slightly larger portions.

Age (years)	Calories (boys)	Calories (girls)
7–10	1,970	1,740
11–14	2,220	1,845

Once children reach the age of 11, their maximum recommended salt intake is the same as an adult's: 6g salt (2.4g sodium) – but remember that this is all too easy to consume, particularly if they eat processed foods.

When they reach puberty (an age that has steadily decreased over the last 100 years), children also have increased requirements for some vitamins and minerals.

Star nutrients for teenagers

Iron

Iron is particularly important, as boys are putting on a lot of muscle at this age, and girls lose iron every month once their periods start. Make sure that your teenager gets plenty of iron-rich foods, such as lean meat (especially red meat), pulses and green vegetables.

If your child shows symptoms of iron deficiency or anaemia, such as tiredness and fatigue, talk to your doctor, as they may need an iron supplement.

Calcium

Calcium is important for all teenagers, as they need to build up their bone density to reduce their risk of the bone-

ANOTHER REASON TO CUT THE FIZZ

Teenagers love fizzy drinks, but they're bad for their bones. Caffeinated drinks, such as cola and energy drinks (and also coffee), can lower body calcium levels. On top of this, the phosphoric acid in fizzy drinks hampers the uptake of bone-building calcium from the diet.

thinning disease osteoporosis when they grow older. This is especially the case for girls, since older women face a higher risk of osteoporosis.

Twenty-five per cent of peak bone mass is acquired during adolescence, but the average teenager's calcium intake is 20% lower than recommended. Dairy products are the main source of calcium in Western countries, but they unfortunately have a rather untrendy reputation among teenagers. Other calcium sources include fish where the bones are eaten (such as tinned salmon or sardines) and tofu (soya bean curd).

Vitamin D

Vitamin D is needed alongside calcium for building bones. The body can make its own vitamin D through the effect of sunlight on the skin, but if your teenager isn't a particularly outdoorsy type, they may not get enough by this route. And this is where diet comes in – you can also get vitamin D from oily fish, milk and eggs.

Healthy fats

The Omega-3 essential fatty acids are particularly important for adolescents, because they're essential for healthy brain development and can help smooth the emotions. And we all know what a rollercoaster teenage moods can be!

And both Omega-3s and the Omega-6s found in nuts and seeds are good for the skin, at a time when this can be a big worry for youngsters.

Fibre

While a high-fibre diet may be a problem for younger children, because it can fill them up before they've eaten enough nutrients, this is rarely an issue for teenagers. Adolescents are more likely to be 'human dustbins' with hearty appetites.

Unfortunately, most teenagers don't eat enough fibre. Surveys show that they prefer white bread to wholemeal, white pasta and rice to brown, and are notoriously bad at eating enough fruit and vegetables. This means you need to steer them away from the refined foods and towards the healthier wholefood versions. Increasing their fibre intake helps keep them full for longer, making them less likely to succumb to unhealthy snacks.

When it comes to persuading teenagers to eat healthily, don't overdo the health angle, unless your child is actually interested. A teenager who thinks you're nagging or 'harping on' about nutrition is likely to rebel, or simply switch off. Teenagers don't generally respond to scare tactics, so telling them they're likely to have a heart attack if they eat fatty foods is unlikely to work. A better tactic is to use the 'what's in it for me?' argument, telling them how healthy eating will help them to have clear skin, glossy hair, good teeth, enhance their sports performance, give them a clear head for passing their exams, and the energy to party!

adapting the plan for very active or sporty children

If your child is very active or does a lot of sports, they may need extra energy and nutrients. If you want to adapt the 6-Week Junk-Free Plan, all you need to do is slightly increase their portion sizes, bearing in mind the following guidance.

Energy

Particularly active children need more calories for 'fuel', and they should get these extra calories from larger portions of healthy carbohydrates (not sugary ones!), and slightly larger protein portions. But don't be tempted to give a sporty child a specially high-protein diet – they don't need it, it doesn't help, and it would unbalance their diet.

Regular refuelling is particularly important for very active children, so be extra strict if they attempt to skip meals, and warn them that this will harm their performance.

Hydration

Active children also need more liquid, to prevent dehydration, because extra fluids are lost during exercise.

Iron

Because iron is needed for transporting oxygen around the body and for building muscle, it's crucial for child athletes.

If your child is using up more iron than they're taking in, they may gradually deplete their iron stores and eventually develop a deficiency, so watch out for iron deficiency symptoms such as tiredness and weakness.

Explain to sporty children how important iron is, and encourage them to eat iron rich foods, such as lean meat (especially red meat), pulses and green vegetables.

adapting the plan for vegetarian children

A good vegetarian diet can be extremely healthy, but a bad vegetarian diet can be disastrous in nutritional terms! If your child decides to go vegetarian by simply cutting out meat, chicken and fish, and living on bread, pasta, eggs, cheese and convenience food, they'll be setting themselves on the road to poor health.

If you're going to feed your child a vegetarian diet, you need to pay particular attention to good nutrition. This is also one of those cases where it might be a good idea to give your child a good-quality multivitamin supplement, just as a kind of 'health insurance' in case they don't hit their nutrient targets all the time.

If you want your vegetarian child to follow the 6-Week Junk-Free Plan, it's not too difficult to avoid the meat and fish options. Just bear in mind the advice below when making your choices, to ensure your child gets all the nutrients they need.

Protein

Obviously, fruit, vegetables and wholegrains are all great vegetarian foods! More problematic is providing good, low-fat sources of protein. Wholegrains contain some protein, but your child needs more.

This is where pulses – beans and lentils – really come into their own! They're filling and nutritious, and contain plenty of vitamins, minerals and phytochemicals.

Products made from soya, Quorn and tofu are also good vegetarian protein sources – but check the label for the salt content, as it can be high in some products.

Eggs and dairy products are good sources of protein, and dairy is great for bone-building calcium, but they can be high in fat. And although they're not meat products (and so are allowable for vegetarians), they're still animal products, and as a rule this means that a high proportion of the fat they do contain will be less-healthy saturated fat.

So, you just want to choose low-fat versions wherever possible. Go for low-fat cheese, low-fat yoghurt, and semi-skimmed or skimmed milk.

To further reduce your vegetarian child's saturated fat intake, use a spread that's high in mono-unsaturates and poly-unsaturates, instead of butter.

VEGGIE 'JUNK FOOD'

Just because the label says it's suitable for vegetarians doesn't mean it has to be healthy. A surprisingly high proportion of manufactured foods marketed for vegetarians are alarmingly high in fat, salt and additives.

They're not *all* bad – you just have to keep your wits about you, so check the labels carefully when buying veggie burgers, grills, vegetarian meat substitutes, and especially vegetarian ready meals.

Nuts are also protein-rich – especially peanuts and cashew nuts (choose the unsalted ones) and walnuts. They're high in healthy unsaturated fats, too. But because even healthy fats are high in calories, you may wish to limit the nuts if you are trying to help your child to lose weight.

Iron

You need to be careful to ensure that your vegetarian child gets enough iron, because the form of iron that's easiest for the body to use is the kind found in meat products. But your child can also get iron from nutritious vegetarian sources – you just need to know where to look!

Good vegetarian sources are dried fruit, (especially apricots), molasses, beans, lentils, egg yolks, wholegrain cereals and green vegetables. Giving your child vitamin C-rich foods at the same time as their iron foods will help them to absorb the iron – try a small glass of orange juice with a meal, or a kiwifruit or some orange segments for dessert.

Vitamin B12

Your child needs vitamin B12 for making healthy red blood cells, and it's found mainly in animal products. If your vegetarian child isn't a big fan of eggs and dairy products (the main non-meat sources), they may become deficient. In this case, it's a good idea to give them a good-quality multivitamin supplement that includes the recommended daily amount of vitamin B12 for children.

Calcium

If your child drinks milk and enjoys other dairy products, getting enough calcium shouldn't be a problem for them. But if you struggle to get dairy inside them, or if they're allergic or intolerant to dairy products, you'll need to find their calcium elsewhere. Good vegetarian sources include tofu, sesame seeds, nuts (especially almonds), dried fruit (especially figs) and green vegetables.

FILLING FIBRE

Vegetarian diets are generally high in fibre. On the one hand, this is a good thing – fibre is good for children's digestion, and it's heart-healthy too. But, if all the fibre in a vegetarian child's diet is filling him or her up before they can finish their meals, consider replacing some of the 'brown' foods such as wholemeal bread, brown rice and brown pasta, with their 'white' alternatives. Don't be tempted to decrease the fruit and vegetables – they may be rich in fibre, but children need all the fruit and veg you can get inside them!

food allergies and intolerances

Sometimes food 'disagrees' with a child. This can be caused by a food allergy, or an intolerance. Food intolerances are less serious than allergies, but can still be very unpleasant and uncomfortable for a child.

Children suffer more from food sensitivities than adults. Between 5% and 8 % of children are thought to suffer from some kind of food sensitivity, compared with 1–2% of adults.

READING THE LABELS

If you discover that your child needs to avoid, for example, all dairy products, or anything containing wheat or nut products, you'll need to become a label sleuth! You might be surprised to learn that, if dairy is 'out', you'll also need to look out for anything containing lactose, whey, milk protein, casein and several others. Don't worry – just talk to your doctor, and they or a dietician will be able to give you a list of all the things you need to avoid.

Allergies

In a true food allergy, the body's immune system launches an over-reaction to the food, causing immediate or almost immediate symptoms such as an itchy mouth, swollen lips, a rash, diarrhoea, vomiting, sneezing, runny nose, and shortness of breath (but fortunately not all of them).

Allergies are much less common than other kinds of food sensitivity, though once again they're seen more frequently in children than adults. Fortunately, though, many of them grow out of it.

The most common food allergies are:

▶▶ Peanuts
▶▶ Other nuts
▶▶ Cows' milk
▶▶ Fish and shellfish
▶▶ Eggs
▶▶ Soya
▶▶ Wheat
▶▶ Kiwifruit

Some children may experience a more severe reaction called anaphylaxis or 'anaphylactic shock' after eating a food they are extremely allergic to. When this happens, the lips and throat can swell, the child can have difficulty in breathing, their blood pressure may suddenly drop and they may even fall unconscious.

Because anaphylactic shock is extremely serious, and can be fatal, if your child suffers from an allergy where anaphylaxis is a risk, your doctor will advise you of the symptoms to look out for, and what to do in such an emergency. Your dietician can advise you on all the foods your child must avoid – it's obvious that a child with a peanut allergy must avoid packets of salted peanuts, but you may not spot groundnut oil mentioned low down on a list of ingredients.

Food intolerances

A food intolerance can cause symptoms that appear hours or even days after the offending food is eaten. These symptoms can include a rash, diarrhoea, bloating, nausea and vomiting and chronic fatigue.

Food intolerances are notoriously hard to diagnose. Because the symptoms don't occur immediately, it's hard to link them with particular trigger foods. And many of the symptoms can be caused by things other than food.

Children can be intolerant of a wide variety of foods, including the list above for allergies, but other common triggers in children include strawberries, citrus fruits, sesame seeds and chocolate.

Probably the best-known food intolerance is one to milk. Fortunately, there are plenty of milk alternatives available, including soya milk, rice milk and oat milk. Children can react to various components in milk, and if lactose (milk sugar) is the problem (lactose intolerance), then lactose-free milk could be the answer.

Some children can't take cows' milk, but can drink goats' milk or ewes' milk without symptoms, so don't assume that all 'animal milk' products will be a problem. You may also find that your cows' milk-intolerant child can eat cows' milk yoghurt and cheese without any ill effects.

Diagnosis

Allergies are diagnosed using skin-prick tests or blood tests, which your doctor can arrange. Intolerances are harder to pin down – you'll need to complete a 'food diary' for your child, noting down everything they eat over a period of time, along with any symptoms, in order to deduce what the problem could be. A dietician or registered nutritionist can then give your child an eating plan that excludes the suspected trigger, to see whether removing that removes the problem. Sometimes it can take a long time and many tries to find the true culprit or culprits!

Be very wary of any tests for food allergies, intolerances and sensitivities offered by alternative practitioners, health food stores and un-registered nutritionists. For an allergy, a doctor is what you need in order to get the correct tests done, and if an intolerance is the problem, he or she can refer you to a registered nutritional professional.

Don't go it alone

If you feel that certain foods may be causing symptoms in your child, it's important for you to take them to see your GP, who can arrange an allergy test if necessary. Don't be tempted to simply cut the offending foods out of their diet. A well-balanced diet is particularly important for growing children, and removing foods or whole food groups from a child's diet could put them at risk of serious nutritional deficiencies.

If your doctor does decide your child has a food sensitivity, he or she can explain to you the various treatments available (in the case of an allergy) and refer you to a registered nutritional professional, such as a dietician, who can ensure that your child receives all the nutrients they need, while avoiding the 'trigger food' or foods.

adapting the 6-week junk-free plan for children with food allergies and intolerances

If your child has a food allergy or intolerance, you'll need to substitute any meals or snacks containing the trigger food, or adapt recipes where you think that the offending food is left out.

If it's practical, it's kinder for the whole family to avoid the trigger food, at least for meals where the child is present. Imagine how frustrating it would be to see everyone else eating the food that you're not allowed!

You need to explain to your child why it's important for them to avoid certain foods, and how to explain to other children and adults why they have to do this. In the case of allergies, particularly the kind that could lead to life-threatening anaphylactic shock, this is especially important, and your school and any clubs your child attends will also need to be told.

In the case of food intolerances, though, it's important that the child doesn't thinking you're making too big a deal of it. You don't want them to think they're on a 'special diet', or that they're missing out on something.

All of the major supermarket chains now produce 'free from' lists of their own brand products, and you can request these from the supermarket's Head Office Customer Services Department.

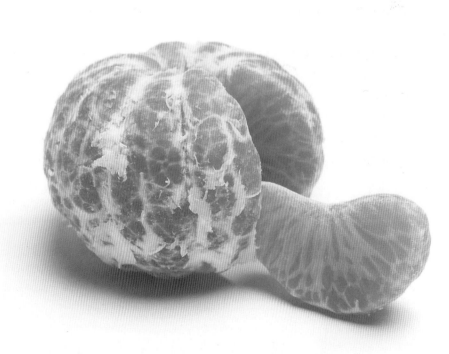

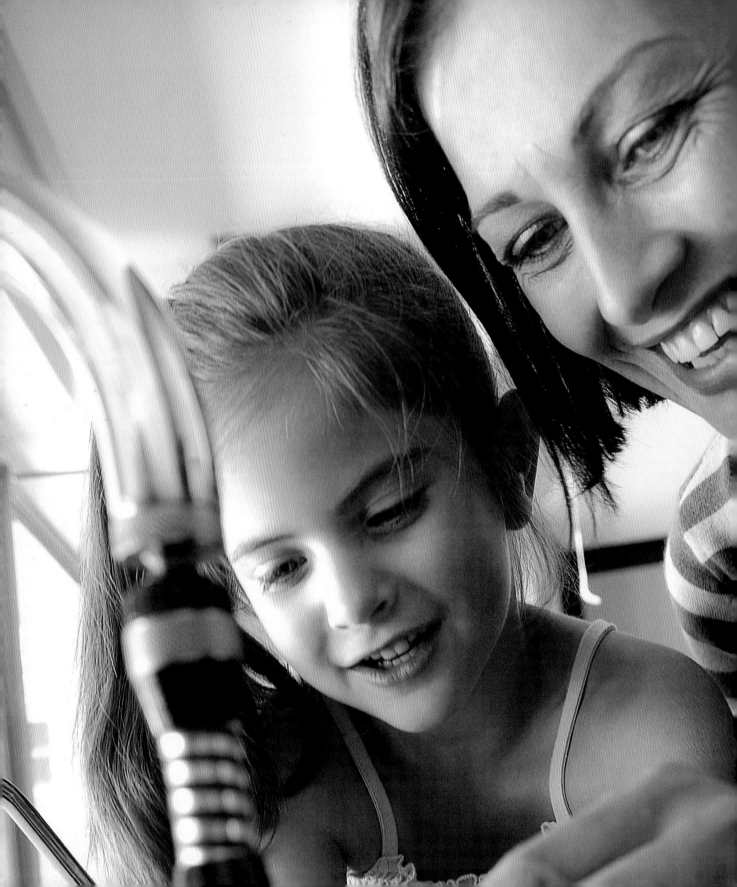

PART 3
MAINTENANCE

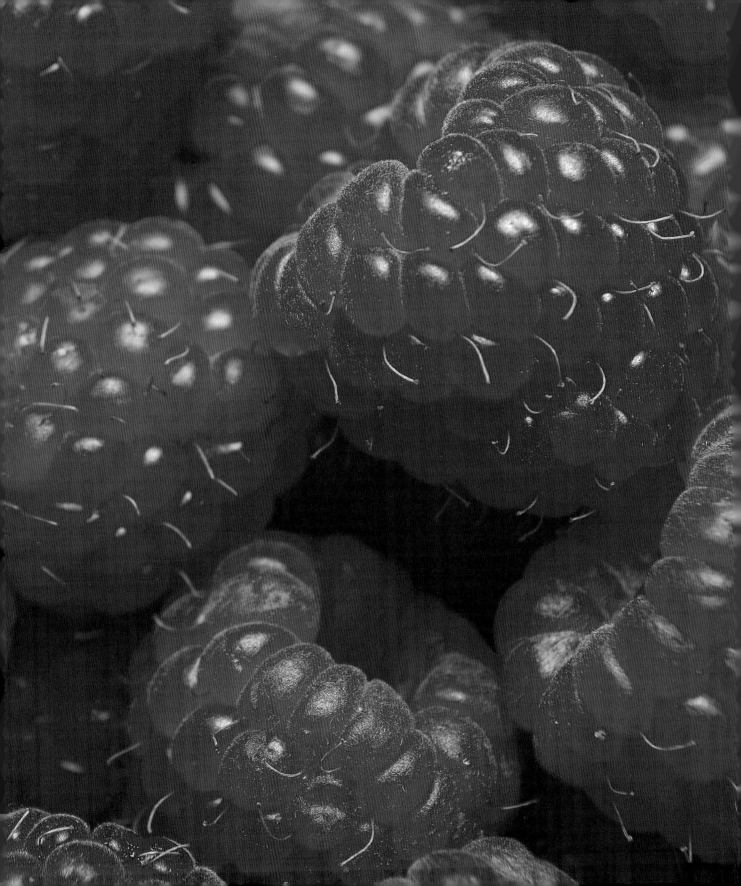

CHAPTER EIGHT

How to Maintain Your Healthy Lifestyle

If you've worked your way through the 6-Week Junk-Free Plan, you're hopefully beginning to see the benefits, in terms of your child's health and happier moods – not to mention your own peace of mind!

But this isn't the end of the story – it's just the beginning. Once your family is junk free – at least most of the time – you can spend more time developing your child's interest in good, nutritious food.

Let them help in the kitchen – children, even very little ones, love cooking.

Teach them how to choose fresh healthy food from the supermarket and, if they're old enough, read labels. Let them grow a few simple vegetables in the garden or herbs on the kitchen windowsill.

Now you're enjoying a whole new way of eating it's time to be a bit more adventurous and add to our plan by devising your own fresh, healthy meals. Take a fresh look at your cookbooks and magazines for healthy recipes you can try and see if any of your old favourites need a nutritional 'facelift'. Could you reduce some of the fat, sugar or salt in any of them? It is so important that we give our children the chance to eat well and to make food fun. I strongly believe that by teaching our kids the basics of cooking and nutrition it will help them for the rest of their lives.

But be realistic. If you eat healthily most of the time, you're allowed to relax sometimes. Even a de-junked family can enjoy the occasional meal in a fast-food restaurant, an ice cream or sticky bun. And the de-junked child needs to know he can 'splurge' at a friend's birthday party without being made to feel guilty.

I don't think you should ban your kids from eating pizzas, crisps or sweets, just don't make them the basis of their diet. It is all too easy to give them processed food and to get a carry out or go to a fast food restaurant, but these should be occasional treats and not a way of life.

'healthify' your favourite recipes

Deciding to revamp your family's diet won't mean you have to abandon all your favourite recipes. But some may need a few tweaks to make them healthier. You'll also find healthier versions of a lot of our old favourites in the Recipes Section in Part 5.

Here are a few simple ways to adapt recipes.

▶▶ Experiment with reducing the amount of sugar used when baking cakes and biscuits. Recipes containing dried fruit often don't need as much sugar as the recipe says – the sweetness in dried fruit is concentrated.

▶▶ Sometimes you can use mashed banana to replace some of the sugar in baking. You'll probably need to use less liquid, as the banana provides moistness.

▶▶ Use soft brown sugar to sweeten desserts. As it has a sweeter taste you will be able to use less.

▶▶ Measure oil into a teaspoon before adding it to a pan, you'll use less than if you pour it straight from the bottle. Or use a spray oil.

▶▶ When stir-frying vegetables use only a teaspoon of oil in the frying pan or wok. Add a little water during cooking to prevent the vegetables from sticking.

▶▶ Make or buy oil-free dressings for salads.

▶▶ Use herbs, spices and seasonings to flavour food and reduce the amount of salt you add during cooking.

creating savvy shoppers

Visits to the shops don't have to be battlegrounds. Children are more likely to enjoy shopping if you involve them in what you are buying. That's not to say they choose what you buy – you don't want a trolley full of cola and crisps! It's got to be you who decides what actually goes into the trolley and what stays on the shelf.

Armed with your trusty shopping list, let them help you to choose the rosiest apples, or the juiciest-looking oranges. As they get older, help them to find the healthiest yoghurts and look at the labels to discover which foods are high in salt, sugar and fat. They'll feel so grown up if they think you are relying on them to help you find the best things to eat!

Children can become anxious and confused if you confront them with a huge range of choices, particularly if they know you're in a hurry to get out of the supermarket. Instead of waving your arm towards a sea of fruit which will seem to them to stretch for miles, simply ask: 'Shall we have these apples or those ones?', or 'would you like the dumpy pears or the long thin ones?' That way they feel they are making the choice but won't be confused by too many options.

Pretend you can't find something inches away from your nose, and ask them to look for it, or set them a task of finding six carrots all about the same size, 10 tiny button mushrooms, or ten nice-looking tomatoes. You could even give them part of the shopping list, just four or five simple items on their own list and make them responsible for finding those items. Children love to feel they are being trusted to do important tasks by adults. As they get older you can give them a list of items needed for the week's school lunchboxes and let them collect those.

The more you can encourage them to take an interest in food, the more likely they are to want to try new foods and to develop into smart shoppers.

Here are just a few shopping savvy tips:

▶▶ Avoid shopping at the busiest times of the day, when the shop will be more crowded.

▶▶ Try not to shop when your child is hungry – they're more likely to be tempted by the things you're trying to steer them away from.

▶▶ If you spot a 'new' fruit or vegetable, tell them it's yummy, and that you've been waiting for ages to have some. It they think you're enthusiastic they won't want to miss out on the chance of trying it.

▶▶ Explain how different fruit and vegetables grow. They'll be fascinated to know that mangoes grow on big trees, grapes grow on vines, and that strawberry plants sit on the ground.

▶▶ When they can read the signs and labels, ask them where different fruit and vegetables have come from, and explain the difference between tropical fruits like bananas and pineapples, and those that grow in cooler countries, like apples and pears. Explain why it's best to look for ones that haven't travelled halfway across the world. If you're lucky you might find something from just up the road.

▶▶ Let them choose the fruit for their packed lunches – they'll be more likely to eat it. Encourage them to pick a wide variety, for example, an orange, an apple, a pear, a banana, and two kiwifruit for another day.

▶▶ Once your child is old enough to read and understand labels, encourage them to find the products with 'real' ingredients in them, such as real fruit in yoghurt, rather than flavourings.

▶▶ Ask your child to help you look for the food with the least salt and fat in. Don't assume that children will be turned off by technical terms like 'saturated fat' – most enjoy learning long words (if only to bamboozle Auntie Gladys next time she comes to visit!).

change the way you cook

Just changing the way you cook can make your meals a lot healthier. Choose these methods, to trim the fat and retain the nutrients.

Grilling

Far better than frying, as it allows the fat in poultry, fish and meat to run off. Grilling is a very versatile method – you can cook vegetables such as mushrooms and tomatoes as well as fillets of fish, sardines, chicken breasts and lean, tender cuts of meat.

Consider getting a ridged griddle pan for use on top of the cooker, or an electric health grill. They're great for cooking meat, poultry and fish and allow the fat to drain away. Children also like the 'stripes' they create on food!

Stewing and casseroling

Ideal for slow cooking of cheaper and less tender cuts of meat. Trim off the fat, brown in a pan wiped with a tiny bit of oil, then add your stock and cook slowly on top of the cooker or in the oven.

Oven roasting

Cook meat, poultry, fish or by simply removing the excess fat from meat, and skin from poultry, spraying the food lightly with olive oil, and cooking open on a rack in a non-stick roaster or in foil parcels. Vegetables can also be oven roasted.

Baked 'parcels'

Bake vegetables, skinned boneless chicken and fish in greaseproof paper parcels. Serve them up still in their wrappings. Children can have their own individual parcel to (carefully – watch out for the steam) open at the table.

Stir-frying

Stir-fries are popular with children, because they're colourful and the vegetables stay crunchy. So get yourself a wok! You only need a quick spray of a good quality oil to create tasty, healthy stir-fries based around vegetables, with lean meat, poultry, prawns, tofu chunks or Quorn for protein. Serve with noodles or rice.

FAT CUTTING TIPS

Rather than putting oil into a pan when you're about to cook something, lightly spray the food (rather than the whole pan). You'll find you can get away with much less oil.

Use low-fat spread on your bread, and go easy! If you're making sandwiches with a moist filling, don't use any spread. You can also cut back by spreading your bread for sandwiches with a reduced fat mayonnaise, salad cream or tomato purée.

Steaming

Get a metal steamer or bamboo steamer basket that fits in your saucepan, or an electric steamer. Vegetables, poultry and fish are all perfect for steaming, and you don't need to add any fat. Steaming is also a great way to retain the vitamins and minerals when cooking vegetables. When you boil food, you lose a lot of the water-soluble vitamins (the B vitamins and vitamin C) into the cooking water.

Poaching

Poaching in water or stock requires no fat. It's ideal for vegetables, chicken, fish and eggs.

timesavers
Make friends with your freezer

Making the most of your freezer (and microwave) makes good sense when you're a busy parent with a family to feed. Having some of their favourite foods stored in the freezer, to be quickly reheated in the oven, on the stove or in the microwave, will save you time and effort, and certainly beats cooking from scratch every single day.

When you're preparing a curry, Bolognese sauce, lasagne or stew, it won't take much longer to cook a double-sized batch and freeze some for a quick meal later. Freezing away batches of homemade basic 'ready-to-use' Pasta Pronto Tomato Sauce (see Recipes Section in Part 5) to pour on pasta is a real time saver, too. You can always ring the changes by adding additional ingredients (such as diced courgettes, thinly sliced mushrooms, peas, sweetcorn, fresh herbs, cooked ham or cooked chicken or grated cheese) to the sauce at the last minute. And it's a great way to get more vegetables into your child's diet.

Freeze sauces in meal-sized portions – it will save you having to attack a large block of frozen sauce to get the required amount.

Make batches of homemade chicken nuggets, burgers (bean, vegetable, turkey, lean beef, chicken, lamb) and freeze them interleaved with cling film, so they're easy to grab from the freezer and defrost quickly. If you make your own burgers using meat or fish, always check with your butcher or on the packet label that it is suitable for home freezing. You must never refreeze raw meat or fish if it has already been frozen. If you have a mincer (or a butcher willing to mince small quantities of meat for you) it might be worth buying cuts of meat rather than ready-minced – that way you can choose leaner meat.

If your family really like their burgers it might be worth investing in a small burger maker – they're simple to use and only cost a few pounds. They come with waxed disks which you put on the top and bottom of the burgers as you press them, making them simple to remove and easy to stack. It also means you can make your burgers actually look like the shop-bought ones – but they'll be much healthier, of course.

If you're a confident cook and occasionally have some time on your hands, look out for some of the less expensive cuts of meat and use them to make nutritious stews and casseroles. These cuts need a little more care in the preparation and take longer to cook, but they really are well worth the effort and freeze well.

Stock up on chicken breasts, thighs (very tasty and ideal for curries and casseroles) and drumsticks, and turkey steaks, when they're on special offer in the supermarket or at the butcher, and freeze them for later.

If you can get to a 'pick-your-own' farm and have room in the freezer, it's worthwhile stocking up on seasonal fruits as they become available. You'll often find that picking your own strawberries, raspberries and blackcurrants is cheaper than buying them in the supermarket, and the children will love joining in.

Other freezer fillers

▶▶ Make or buy pizza bases to whip out of the freezer and finish off with a healthy topping.

▶▶ Stock up on wholewheat chapattis and wheat or corn tortillas to make 'wraps' and enchiladas.

▶▶ Frozen peas and sweetcorn – perfect when you need a quick vegetable as an accompaniment, or to add to other dishes.

▶▶ Fillets of white fish or salmon to bake for a quick lunch or supper.

▶▶ Have a pack of wholemeal pitta breads in the freezer –

they're great for a quick snack. Split the pittas in half and toast or warm in the oven. They're ideal to dip into yoghurt-based dips or low-fat hummus, along with vegetable sticks.

kids in the kitchen

Some of my happiest memories of growing up are helping my mum in the kitchen, and she says it made the chore of cooking meals much more enjoyable too.

Getting children involved in the kitchen is an important – and fun – way of giving them the know-how to help them to make good food choices. If they get used to seeing ingredients in their raw state at home, they're less likely to grow up thinking that meals appear ready-made from boxes and cartons.

You certainly don't need to have formal cooking sessions or lessons, for a start just let them help to prepare family meals. Give them simple jobs to begin with like topping a pizza, even if it's only selecting the toppings or sprinkling on the cheese.

Even quite young children can become surprisingly accomplished little chefs if they're given the chance to gain confidence in the kitchen. By the time they reach their teens they should be able to cook simple healthy meals for themselves and will hopefully be less likely to reach for a ready-meal.

Helping you to make a few fairy cakes, some simple bread, a lunchbox cereal bar, some muffins or a batch of homemade burgers for the freezer are great activities for a wet Saturday afternoon when they can't get out to play. Keep cooking sessions short, or they'll become bored and you'll be

left to finish the job. Cooking is also the perfect way to teach them kitchen hygiene, safety and the need to tidy up when they've finished a job!

Safety first

You know your child better than anyone, so use your judgement to decide when it is safe for them to handle sharp knives and other pieces of kitchen equipment.

Here are just a few safety rules you'll need to teach them:

▶▶ Never run in the kitchen.
▶▶ Always dry your hands carefully before touching anything electric.
▶▶ Never hold ingredients in your hands when cutting them – cut them on a chopping board.
▶▶ Never put sharp knives into the washing up bowl – someone might put their hands into the soapy water and cut themselves.
▶▶ Never put your hands in a food processor or blender when it is switched on (most have safety guards and cut-out devices to prevent this, but older models may not).
▶▶ Always use oven gloves to take hot dishes from the oven or microwave.
▶▶ Stand well back from gas burners as you switch them on and remember that an electric hob remains hot for some time after it is switched off.
▶▶ Remember to turn of the cooker, oven or grill when you have finished cooking.
▶▶ Never leave a hot pan or frying pan unattended, particularly if it contains oil.

PACK A PICNIC AND HEAD FOR THE PARK:

If the weather is fine think of having a picnic ... Not the smoked salmon, strawberries and champagne variety, just a simple meal that your child can help to prepare, popped into a coolbag, to enjoy under a shady tree in the local park or even in the garden. All you need is a few small sandwiches, a homemade biscuit or cake, a piece of fruit and a drink.

And a few basic hygiene rules:

▶▶ Always wash your hands before beginning to cook, and again after touching, meat, fish or poultry.

▶▶ Always wash fruit and vegetables before cooking or eating them.

▶▶ Always cut meat, fish, and vegetables on separate chopping boards.

▶▶ If you take food out of the fridge, don't leave it sitting around to get warm if it's not to be eaten straight away. Put it back in the fridge as soon as possible.

Jobs for junior cooks

Here's a guide to some of the tasks children may be able to manage at different ages. You are the best judge of what your child is capable of, but always err on the side of safety and don't let children undertake tasks unless you are confident they will be able to manage them. And always supervise.

3–6-Year-Olds

▶▶ Counting and washing fruit and vegetables

▶▶ Cutting out shapes with cookie cutters

▶▶ Placing biscuits on a cold baking sheet

▶▶ Mixing cold ingredients in a bowl

6–10-Year-Olds

▶▶ Reading simple recipes

▶▶ Writing shopping lists

▶▶ Preparing some vegetables (for example removing outer leaves from sweetcorn, shelling peas, removing hulls from strawberries, peeling and crushing garlic)

▶▶ Measuring and weighing dry ingredients

▶▶ Measuring liquid ingredients into a jug

▶▶ Using a blunt knife for spreading

10–12-Year-Olds

▶▶ Following a simple recipe with a little supervision

▶▶ Using a hob, oven or microwave with a little supervision

▶▶ Using a hand electric mixer

OR HAVE AN AFTER-SCHOOL FRUITNIC:

If you have some spare time after collecting them from school, head for the nearest park or play area with a box filled with pieces of fruit, a healthy biscuit and a drink. Just giving the children half an hour to unwind and share any worries of the day, will mean you all arrive home more relaxed.

▶▶ Using a hand grater (not a mandolin)

▶▶ Using a sharp knife with supervision

Teenagers

By the time they're teenagers, if they have been taught to cook from a young age, most youngsters will be ready to plan and prepare a healthy meal and write their own shopping list. They will also be able to use a wide variety of kitchen equipment, like the food processor and blender, safely. Hopefully they will also enjoy cooking, and it'll stand them in good stead when they go away to college or leave home!

dig this!

Children love growing things, so make the most of their enthusiasm. Whether it's just a few herbs in pots on the windowsill, cress on some damp kitchen towel on a saucer, some sprouting seeds or a full-blown vegetable plot, they'll be fascinated by watching them grow. We have a tub outside the kitchen full of herbs which we planted together and we use in cooking. Everything really does taste so much nicer when you pick it fresh from the plant.

Even if your fingers are not even the palest shade of green, it's still possible and actually fun to grow a few of your own vegetables and some fruit. It's not rocket science and you don't need a large garden or even a special vegetable plot. You'll be surprised how much you can grow in a few old containers, troughs and pots, or you might even have a fruit tree or two in your garden – if so, make the most of it! And there's nothing to stop you dotting the odd vegetable or soft fruit plant in among the flower beds. If you put the veggies and fruit at or near the front of the beds, your child can hunt

BAKING BREAD

Making bread is really simple and all that kneading and shaping and watching it rise is great fun for children. And let them work out their pent-up energy and frustration by punching and kneading the dough! If you use a complete bread mix it's not as laborious as you may think – all you have to do is add water. There are only a couple of periods of actual breadmaking 'work', with long breaks in between to let the dough rise and do its stuff!

There are a wide variety of bread mixes available in the supermarket from plain white and wholemeal to multigrain, fruit, tomato, onion, and even some of the Continental favourites like ciabatta. Look for mixes that don't contain hydrogenated fats.

If you have a breadmaker you can speed up the process by using the dough setting and removing the dough for the shaping and final rise. One thing's for sure – children won't be able to resist tasting the bread when it comes out of the oven.

them out among the flowers when it's time to harvest them without damaging any precious blooms.

You can also get a good crop of new potatoes by planting a few tubers in a black garden rubbish sack with a few holes in the bottom, to prevent them from getting waterlogged.

All you need to get started is some good garden soil or

compost and a few tools – what you need will depend on how adventurous you plan to be. If you're only going to plant a few containers or pots, and dot fruit and veg in the flower beds, it'll just be a strong trowel, a watering can, and perhaps a few short bamboo canes and some garden string if anything needs a little support.

Obviously, start off with the simple vegetables and fruits (leave celery and asparagus to the experts!) and those which grow quickly – to allow for child-sized attention spans. Waiting for most seeds to germinate can seem like an eternity to children so if you want to speed things up pick up small trays of lettuce plants, beetroot, peas, courgettes, cabbage, sprouting broccoli or cauliflower from the garden centre and just transplant them into your garden.

Another good idea is to pick up a couple of bush tomato or cherry tomato plants, and perhaps a pepper or aubergine, from the garden centre and grow them in large pots in a sunny spot on the patio.

Radishes, carrots, spring onions and some varieties of lettuce germinate quite quickly, though, so it's worth trying to grow them from seed.

Here are some simple fruit and vegetables you and your children might like to try growing. If you haven't got a garden, all of these (except sweetcorn) are easy to grow in pots, tubs or troughs on a patio or balcony. Once you've grown your own fruit and vegetables, you'll be hooked.

Strawberries

You can grow these in the garden, in pots, or in a special strawberry planter (but pots and planters do tend to dry out very quickly and need more attention). As the strawberries form, place a little straw or a special collar (from the garden centre) under the plants to keep the fruit off the ground – this stops them from rotting. Garden strawberries are irresistible – they're much tastier and sweeter than shop-bought ones.

Peas

Peas don't have to be grown in long rows in allotments – they can be grown in the garden just like sweet peas. You can hang some pea netting from your fence and plant the peas at the base. Or how about letting your child help you to put up a wigwam of bamboo canes, or even grow two peas up a single cane? Just tie the young plants to the canes and watch them grow. It's unlikely, unless you grow loads of them, that many of your home-grown peas will actually find their way into the saucepan – few children can resist eating the sweet tender peas straight from the pod!

French or dwarf beans

These come in several varieties and the pods can be white, yellow, green or black (though they all turn green when you

> ## GOOD PLANTS FOR FLOWER BEDS
>
> All of these pretty fruit and vegetable plants are quite happy to live with the roses, petunias and daisies:
> - **Dwarf beans**
> - **Radishes**
> - **Lettuces**
> - **Strawberries**

cook them, which fascinates most children). You can grow them easily from seed or you can pick up young plants from the garden centre. Look for a heavy-cropping variety and plant them in the flower beds or in containers and troughs. Unless your garden is very windy they won't need any support and will grow as compact and attractive little bushes – which, unlike runner beans, don't need tall people to pick them!. The red or white flowers are very pretty, too. Pick the beans when they are young and lightly boil or steam them to retain their nutrients.

Radishes

These are really simple for children to grow themselves. Just scatter a few seeds into a pot and cover with a light covering of soil. Water gently. When the seedlings appear, thin them out so that the radishes have room to grow big and fat.

Carrots

Pick one of the round varieties (like little golf balls) or a short, stumpy kind. Simply plant two rows in a trough or in the garden and wait for them to germinate. Thin them out to two inches apart and just wait for them to grow. There's nothing nicer than pulling a carrot, rinsing it under the tap and munching it with the green still attached.

Lettuces

You can often pick up a variety of young lettuce plants from the garden centre, so why not grow several different kinds to bring some variety to your salads? Lettuces grow very quickly so you can be eating them a few weeks after planting.

Cut-and-come-again salad and spinach leaves

You can now buy packets of seeds to grow 'cut-and-come-again' mixed salad and baby spinach leaves.

All you have to do is plant the seeds in containers or troughs according to the packet instructions and then, when they're big enough, just gently pull off a few leaves from each plant at a time, to add to salads. If you stagger your planting you can have leaves to cut all summer. Older children often like being given the job of harvesting the day's salad leaves.

Courgettes

These are really easy to grow. Either plant seeds in containers or buy young plants. Pick the courgettes when they are only a few inches long, when they're at their most tender.

Potatoes

If you haven't got space to grow them in the garden, get a few black garden refuse sacks and grow early new potatoes in these. Roll the bags down until they are about eight inches tall and fill them with good garden soil or a multi-purpose compost (you can often pick this up in bags in the supermarket). Plant three new potato tubers into the soil in the bag. As the 'green tops' grow, gradually add more soil until your potato bag is about 14 inches tall. You don't need to harvest all of your potatoes at once. Simply scrabble in the earth gently and lift out enough for a meal, and let the plant continue to grow and more potatoes develop.

Sweetcorn

You might see these at the garden centre – you can often buy six or eight plants in a tray. If you've got a space in the garden, these are well worth growing, but remember, they grow tall. They are a really attractive plant and children will love watching the cobs develop with their long whiskers and green jackets.

Remember even plants welcome a little TLC. Get some liquid organic feed and add it to the water in your watering can when you water your plants. Always follow the instructions and make sure that you always keep the container out of children's reach.

Getting the best from your homegrown harvest

One of the fantastic things about homegrown fruit and vegetables is that you get them as fresh as they can be, with 100% of their nutrients – and zero 'food miles'!

So, you'll want to make sure that you eat them at their best, to maximise the goodness.

▶▶ Eat your harvest as fresh as possible.

▶▶ If they can be eaten raw, eat them this way.

▶▶ Don't overcook your vegetables and always prepare and cook them at the last minute.

▶▶ Store your harvested vegetables in the salad crisper in the fridge, and avoid putting them into plastic bags. Potatoes need to be stored in paper bags in the dark.

If you can't grow your own

If you aren't able to grow your own vegetables, you can still try to get your children familiar with a wide variety of them by letting them see them, touch them and smell them in their 'natural' state, for example corn on the cob, still with its 'whiskers' and green leafy 'wrapping'. Once children's

JOBS FOR JUNIOR GARDENERS

- Helping to choose the seeds or young plants from the shop or garden centre
- Making a little 'drill' with their finger for planting carrot, radish or lettuce seeds
- Planting large, easy-to-handle seeds, such as courgettes, peas and beans
- Planting potatoes in black 'sacks'
- Watering is a fun, easy job that even young children can manage. Explain to them water is especially important for baby plants (though they mustn't be 'drowned'!), so they need regular 'drinks' for the first few weeks until they are well established
- Harvesting, or helping with the harvest – probably the most fun of all!

curiosity is aroused, they'll be more likely to want to try them. It's a sad fact that many children don't even realise that carrots come out of the ground, covered with earth and with feathery tops and that peas grow like rows of identical soldiers in a pod.

If you are out for a drive and come across a 'pick your own' grower or a farm shop, pop in and let your child see what vegetables and fruit look like straight from the fields rather than in polythene bags or plastic trays. It's a good opportunity to be able to talk to them about vegetables and fruit – ask if there's something they'd like to buy to take home to try.

SHOUT FOR SPROUTS

Sprouting seeds is instant gardening and they're full of nutrients.

If you think about it, a sprout contains all of the nutrients and energy needed to make a small seed grow into a plant. So it's no surprise that they're good for us.

There aren't many other seeds that grow into edible plants in a few days, so sprouts are an ideal gardening starter for children – they'll be able to grow and eat several crops while they wait for other seeds to germinate.

Sprouts come in many varieties, from mild to hot, nutty to spicy, and there's a range of ways to use them. Add them to salads, stir-fries, soups, dips, casseroles and stews, or just nibble them on their own. Chinese bean sprouts (mung beans), alfalfa, lentils, broccoli, lentils and chick peas are a few varieties worth trying.

To sprout, all seeds need is water and air. To start sprouting all you need is a wide-necked jam jar, a piece of muslin or fine cotton and an elastic band. It couldn't be simpler.

Health-food shops and garden centres sell packets of seeds for sprouting and a packet will give you many crops as you only use a few seeds at a time. They all come with their own instructions. Just stick to one variety per jar, as they have different germination times – tiny seeds such as alfalfa are faster than big ones like chick peas.

out and about with children

When you're out with your child, you generally have less control over when, where and – most importantly – what they eat.

Normal meal routines are disrupted because you're busy doing other things, and it's easy for your healthy intentions to fly out of the window with all the distractions.

This is when pester power can really kick in. Children can get argumentative and whiney when they're tired and hungry – and who can blame them? And who can blame any parent (probably tired and hassled themselves) from giving in to their little one's demands for chocolate, fizzy drinks, fast food or whatever it was they wanted.

It's better to not let them get to that state in the first place. If you plan ahead, and keep them well-fuelled with healthy, energy providing food, the situation won't arise.

Planning ahead

If you know you're going to be away from home for a meal, you have plenty of options:

▶▶ Take a packed lunch for each person
▶▶ Make it a 'picnic day', with a hamper or chilled backpack of food for everyone to share
▶▶ Find a restaurant, takeaway or shop where you can buy healthy food – more about that later...

Ensure that you've brought plenty of water for everyone to drink.

Taking Control Of Timing

If your child goes too long without food, their blood sugar levels will fall and they'll get hungry, tired and cranky. But you need to be careful what you give them. Sweets, chocolates and fizzy drinks will send their blood sugar levels through the roof. They'll get an instant shot of energy, but that energy hit won't last. All too soon their blood sugar levels will fall again, and they'll be feeling woozy or irritable, and wanting more sugary snacks. And if you give in to their pleas, you set the whole vicious cycle going again!

What do you do? You need to keep their blood sugar levels balanced, with the 'slow-release' kinds of fuels that we've mentioned before.

You need to:

▶▶ Encourage your child to eat something as close as possible to their normal meal time.

▶▶ If you know you're not going to be able to find somewhere to sit down and eat, bring a healthy snack that they can eat on the move, to tide them over until the next proper meal.

▶▶ Make sure that all meals and snacks are 'slow-release' foods, rather than high in sugar.

▶▶ If it's practical, they should carry their own water bottle. They're more likely to take frequent drinks and stay well hydrated if they don't keep having to ask you for a drink.

kids in the car

'Are we there yet?' It's a familiar cry, isn't it? Driving with children can be stressful at the best of times, and it can be all too tempting to keep a child in the back seat quiet with a big bag of sweets or some crisps. But filling them up with food that's full of sugar and fat could prove even worse for your stress levels – and here's why!

Sweets, chocolates and fizzy drinks will send their blood sugar levels soaring, at a time when their mealtime routine is likely as not mixed up, and they're already excited – just the time when you want to be keeping their blood sugar levels (and therefore their energy levels) nice and stable. The child will love that 'sugared-up' feeling, but do you really want them bouncing around the car with all that pent-up energy?

And here comes the crunch. When, all too soon, the energy buzz passes, they'll get cranky and irritable, and want more sugary snacks, leaving the way wide open to set up that whole vicious cycle again.

Instead, you need to keep their blood sugar levels nice and stable. If your child needs a snack to keep him or her going until the next meal, it should be something that's high enough in energy to sustain them, but low in fat and sugar, without any of the additives that many children react to.

Give them fruit (fresh or dried) – it's sweet, but the fibre makes it a 'slow-release fuel', so it's far healthier than sweets. Or offer a homemade (healthy) baked bar or flapjack (see Recipes Section in Part 5), rather than chocolate.

A little bit of protein – such as a cold veggie sausage, or a small pot of nuts and seeds – is another healthy travel snack for a child, and the protein content helps them to feel satisfied and contented.

> **Choose easy-to-eat foods that won't give you a car full of crumbs or sticky hands and faces.**

Six great travel snacks for children

▶▶ Pots of prepared fruit (apple slices, grapes, orange segments, banana. Add a squeeze of lemon juice to stop them from going brown).

▸▸ Oatcakes, mini rice cakes or wholewheat crackers.

▸▸ Vegetable strips (pepper, carrots, cucumber and celery, or even cooked baby new potatoes).

▸▸ Small bags of unsalted nuts and seeds (peanuts, Brazil nuts, almonds, sunflower and pumpkin seeds), or dried fruit, or a mixture of the two.

▸▸ Plain, home-popped popcorn (no salt or sugar)

▸▸ Healthy homemade baked bars or flapjacks (see Recipes Section in Part 5)

healthy eating out

What about if it's not possible or practical to bring your own packed meal – or you simply fancy eating out?

It's perfectly possible to feed your child well when you're away from home. You just need to know the healthy options, and steer your child towards these.

Coffee shops

Coffee shops are popping up in our high streets like mushrooms, and can be a good place for a re-fuelling stop.

If you find one that serves fresh, homemade soup, you're on to a winner! Add a wholemeal roll, and you've got a perfect meal.

A sandwich, ciabatta or wrap makes a good meal, so long as you check the calorie, saturated fat and salt content – some are scarily high.

If there's fresh fruit on the counter, or ready prepared fruit salad, go for this as a dessert.

While you enjoy a cappuccino or skinny latte (treat yourself!), coffee and other highly caffeinated drinks aren't a great idea for children.

If they're happy with water with their meal, breathe a silent sigh of relief! Otherwise, steer your child away from sugary fizzy drinks and milkshakes, and towards drinks such as fresh fruit juice (ask for a glass of water as well, so you can dilute it). If 'fruit juice drink' or low-calorie fizz is all that's available (or that they'll drink), let them – it's only very occasionally, after all.

What about all those sticky cakes and pastries? Try to steer your child past them, or if they notice, wrinkle your nose and call them 'sickly sweet'. But if your child has been eating healthily otherwise, there's nothing wrong with an occasional treat – just choose wisely. Buy them a fruit scone, a currant bun or a teacake and they might think it's sweet enough and doesn't need jam, or suggest a savoury scone with some 'healthy' spread. And a shortbread biscuit, cookie or biscotti is allowable as a treat.

If the sticky cakes and pastries are all there is, buy one between you, and make a fun family thing out of sharing it. Ask for a knife to cut it into little pieces, or ask for a spoon for everyone if it's a 'gooey' cake.

Sandwich bars

Sandwich bars, where your food is prepared in front of you, can be a great place for you and your child to eat, since you can tailor your sandwich, wrap, salad or whatever however you like.

Follow these tips for the healthiest sandwiches in town!

▸▸ Choose wholemeal bread, unless you find it fills your child up too much.

▸▸ Go without spread if the filling is moist.

▸▸ Avoid fillings with mayo, and instead go for those with

low-fat dressings such as salad cream or yoghurt dressings.

▶▶ Low-fat cream cheese is great with cold meat, removing the need for mayo.

▶▶ Ask the assistant to pile in the salad!

Many sandwich bars also sell salad boxes, where they fill up a little plastic tray from a selection of salads.

Tips for healthy salad boxes:

▶▶ Ask what dressings are on each of the salads – look for undressed ones, or those with only a little of a light dressing made from healthy oils such as olive oil.

▶▶ Avoid mayonnaise if at all possible.

▶▶ Include some protein – meat, chicken or turkey, fish such as tuna or salmon (though beware the mayo!) or beans.

▶▶ Plus some carbohydrate – pasta or rice, or buy a bread roll to eat with your salad.

▶▶ Then fill up with a tasty and colourful mix of salad leaves, grated carrot, beetroot, cucumber, pepper, sweetcorn and whatever else is available!

Let your child choose their own salads, once you've established which ones they can choose from. If this is too limiting, let them have a little bit of the less healthy ones, but fill up most of the box with the better options (have a quiet word with the assistant!).

Department store and supermarket cafés

These are getting better. If you walk past the often cooked-to-death hot meals, sweltering under the heat lamps, hopefully you'll be able to find some soup and a crusty roll, or a crisp salad with lean meat, fish or cottage cheese. Or choose a 'healthy option' pre-packed sandwich, wrap or ciabatta, or a baked potato with cottage cheese or baked beans – steer clear of the mayonnaise-covered prawns and the coleslaw.

What about the pick-and-mix 'kids' meals' you often see in these cafés? Children love the colourful cardboard lunchboxes, especially if they contain some colouring pencils and paper, or a toy. And anything that keeps them out of mischief while you enjoy your meal has got to be a welcome treat for you too! Nutritionally, these meals can be good – or dire – depending on the selection of items available, and what you and your child choose.

Good choices include:

▶▶ Sandwiches with low-fat fillings, preferably with some protein such as lean meat or chicken, or egg, and plenty of salad.

▶▶ Fresh fruit.

▶▶ Small boxes of raisins.

▶▶ A matchbox-sized chunk of cheese.

▶▶ 'Cheese dippers' – these aren't a terribly healthy choice to include regularly in lunchboxes, but are OK once in a while.

▶▶ A child-sized currant bun.

▶▶ A small carton of milk.

▶▶ Pure fruit juice (ask for a glass of water to dilute it with).

▶▶ Yoghurt or fromage frais (so long as it's not too high in sugar and/or additives).

Steer clear of:

▶▶ Crisps

▶▶ Chocolate bars

▶▶ Sweets

▶▶ Fruit juice drinks

▶▶ Fizzy drinks

Pizza places

The healthiest option is for your child to have a healthy main meal salad – some pizza chains have 'self-serve' salad bars, which are great. If your child is old enough to serve themselves, you can point out the healthy options that you're happy for them to have, and then let them decide how much of each thing they have. Encourage them to include some beans or pulses for protein, some potato salad or pasta salad for carbohydrate, and then pile the rest of the plate high with yummy, fresh salad. Steer them away from the creamy dressings! If they don't fancy potato salad or pasta salad, suggest that they have a side helping of potato wedges, to fill them up. They're fried, but do contain some fibre in the skins. But avoid the garlic bread and fried onion rings – they really are fat traps!

Many children will make a bee-line for the pizza menu. When you order, go for a thin and crispy rather than a deep pan or cheese-stuffed crust. Give the pizzas topped with meat or sausage a miss, and choose prawns, pineapple and vegetables instead. And ask the waiter to go easy on the cheese!

Burger bars and other fast-food chains

Many burger restaurants are smartening up their act, with low-fat options – so you can feed your child healthily, if you know what to choose. Fortunately, many of the fast-food chains are proud of their healthier items, and you can pick up leaflets showing the calories, fat, sugar and salt in your meal. Make a point of reading these, to avoid any nasty nutritional surprises!

Try to persuade your child to have grilled chicken or fish fingers, with a salad, rather than a burger, cheeseburger, chickenburger or battered chicken with fries. Even healthy-sounding veggie-burgers can be as high in fat as a beefburger – see if the burger chain produces a nutritional leaflet, and check before you buy. If your little one digs their heels in, suggest a compromise. How about grilled chicken with fries? Or a burger with a salad? One little tip – watch out for high-fat creamy dressings with the salad, or you could end up eating as much fat than if you'd had the fries!

Drinks can be a nutritional minefield. A child with a large fizzy drink can be gulping down nearly 250 calories and 11 teaspoons of sugar. Thick shakes are even worse, with over 500 calories, 13g of fat and 16 teaspoons of sugar. Slurp, slurp, slurp, and that's nearly half of their recommended maximum fat allowance, around a third of their calories, and approximately one-and-a-third times *more* than their recommended sugar allowance for the whole day!

But when all is said and done, if the only alternative to all-out war is to relent and give in to the burger and fries option, then do so and don't worry about it. One less-than-healthy meal isn't going to harm them. Just resolve not to bring them to this particular restaurant next time you're out!

Shop-bought sandwiches and lunches

A shop-bought sandwich can be a good lunch on the move, but you need to check the label, as some can tot up an amazing 750 calories – nearly half of a child's recommended total. Thankfully more and more healthy options are appearing in supermarket chiller cabinets and sandwich bars. Check the labels for calories, salt and fat (especially saturated fat) – anything with mayonnaise or creamy dressing will be sky high. Ploughman's, and most other sandwiches with cheese, are also high.

Choose a sandwich with some low-fat protein – fish, lean meat, poultry or low-fat cheese – with plenty of salad and a low-fat dressing.

A shop-bought pasta salad is another healthy choice for children, so long as you check the fat content – sometimes the dressings are very oily. Also try to go for one that has plenty of vegetables in.

Or try one of those little takeaway sushi boxes you can buy from the supermarkets nowadays. Their 'grown-up-ness', not to mention the fact that they look quirky and fun, will appeal to most children. Sushi is also low in fat, and the rice is a good source of complex carbohydrate.

dining out

'Dining out', whether it's lunch during a shopping trip, or a birthday celebration, is a great treat for children. It's a good way for them to try new foods, and to learn how to behave and eat politely in public. And best of all – you don't have a mountain of washing up afterwards!

Restaurants are getting more 'child-friendly', and most will accommodate slight changes to their menu, if you ask nicely and explain that it's for the little one. Ask if they'll do a smaller portion, perhaps served 'plainer', without the sauce. If only more restaurants did this! Don't be fobbed off with a restaurant that offers a special 'children's menu' of fish and chips, baked beans and chicken nuggets, while the adults enjoy finer fare! Why shouldn't children have the same as you?

Chinese restaurants

Many children adore Chinese food – it's generally brightly coloured, sweet tasting and fun to eat! Unfortunately, it can be high in fat, sugar and monosodium glutamate (MSG), which many children (and adults) can have a bad reaction to.

A Chinese meal or takeaway is fine once in a while, just steer your child towards one of the following:

▶▶ Steamed or stir-fried dishes
▶▶ Plain boiled or steamed rice
▶▶ Vegetable, prawn, or chicken dishes, rather than duck or beef

Avoid, or buy just one portion to share between all of you:

▶▶ Anything that's called 'crispy' – it's deep fried in batter
▶▶ Anything that even mentions batter
▶▶ Fried rice
▶▶ Prawn toasts
▶▶ Spring rolls

Indian restaurants

Indian food tends to be either very healthy – or very heavy and oily.

Steer your child towards:

▶▶ Plain boiled or steamed rice
▶▶ Tikka or tandoori dishes (not tikka massala – this is tremendously high in fat)
▶▶ Salads
▶▶ Chapattis

Avoid, or buy just one portion to share between all of you:

▶▶ Curries, particularly the creamy ones, such as korma and passanda
▶▶ Pilau rice – it's high in fat, while plain rice is fat-free
▶▶ Onion bhajis and pakoras
▶▶ Sticky, deep-fried desserts

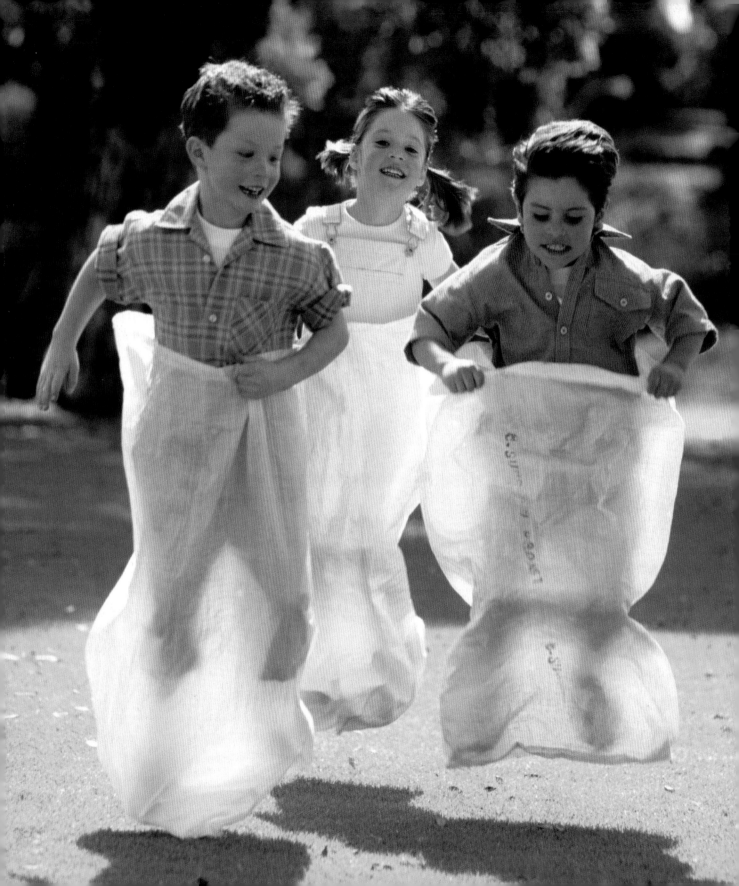

PART 4
ACTIVITY AND EXERCISE

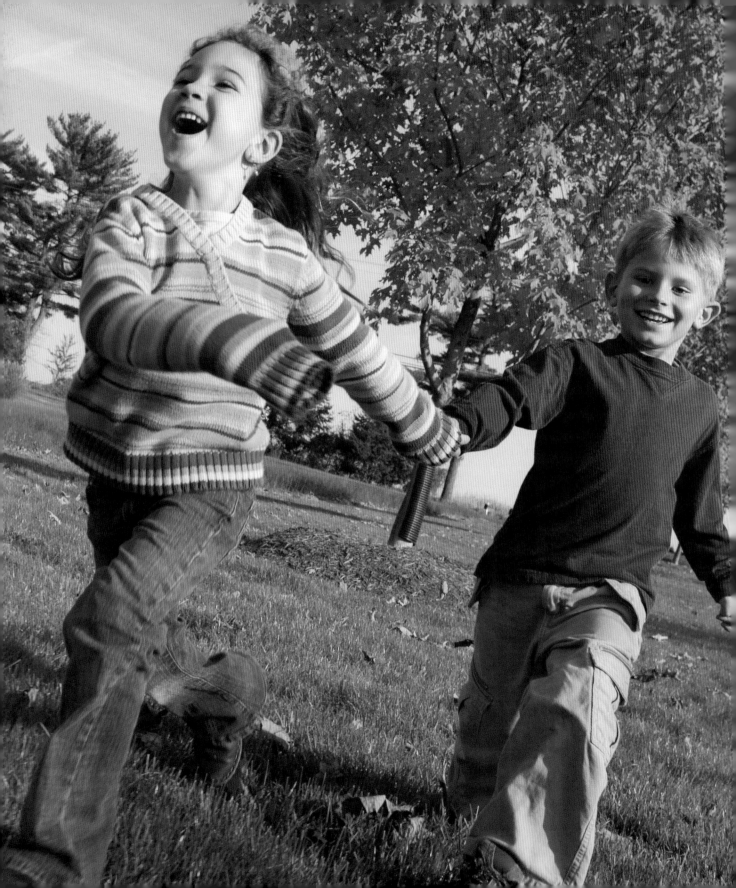

CHAPTER NINE

ACTIVITY AND EXERCISE

Nutritious food is only part of the equation for happy, healthy children – they also need exercise to help them live life to the full.

Children are built for running about. This, rather than computer games and television, is what their young bodies are crying out for.

They just need encouragement – exercise is fun!

It's also positively healthy. Exercise builds strong bones and muscles, is good for children's blood pressure and cholesterol levels, supports the immune system and improves their co-ordination and flexibility.

But it also has some other benefits that might not be so obvious. All that running around – particularly if it's out in the fresh air – builds up a healthy appetite, and helps children to sleep well at night. Exercise helps prevent them from getting stressed by allowing them to 'let off steam'. It also teaches children the value of practice and teamwork, and how to be good winners and losers.

And of course, exercise plays a vital role in preventing children from putting on weight.

how much exercise?

The official recommendation is for children to have at least an hour of 'moderate physical activity' each day – and this really isn't that difficult to achieve.

Tips for sneaking activity into a child's day

All of these will help keep your child fit and burn up energy.

▶▶ Kicking a ball around
▶▶ Riding a bike, either with friends or on family bike rides (make sure you have the right safety equipment)

▶▶ Skipping

▶▶ Playing with 'active' toys

▶▶ Throwing a Frisbee

▶▶ Skateboarding

▶▶ Helping to exercise the dog

▶▶ Dancing

▶▶ Helping with housework

▶▶ Gardening

▶▶ Running around during school playtime

▶▶ Walking to school (if it's safe and practical)

▶▶ Helping with the shopping

sporty children

There's no such thing as a child who 'doesn't like sport'. You just have to find activities that suit their personality and abilities.

No child likes to look silly, so if they simply can't get the hang of tennis, or they loathe running, don't push the issue.

It may be that their bodies simply aren't built to be good at that particular sport. For example, although you don't have to be tremendously tall to enjoy and benefit from playing basketball, a short child may feel out of place on a team of lanky beanpoles!

Of course, some children love a challenge, and if your child asks to try a sport they don't seem to be cut out for, you shouldn't prevent them from having a go at it.

Ask your child for suggestions – they may have a deep down longing to try an activity you'd never thought of, like yoga, archery, or skateboarding!

And if your child says they're no good at sport, they're probably just being modest! Have a word with their PE

> Make sure that your child's sport is related to their own interests, not yours. You may have been the star of your school hockey team, or adored horseriding – but your child could hate it!

teacher and ask where your child's talents lie – they may have spotted an aptitude that your child hasn't noticed.

A graceful child could be encouraged in activities such as drama, dance and gymnastics; a strong, powerful child may have great potential for athletics, and one with great hand-to-eye coordination could be encouraged to try cricket or tennis.

Sadly, some children find school PE lessons a miserable experience – trying and failing with all your friends watching can be embarrassing and discouraging. If your child is struggling with PE at school, you might be able to help. Practise with them, for example kicking a ball for a young goalie to save, buying a netball hoop so they can practise their shooting technique, or helping them to practise their batting and fielding skills at rounders or cricket in the park. Even something as simple as playing catch together can help with hand-to-eye coordination.

In a less threatening situation, with support and encouragement from you, they may be able to relax and perform better, building their confidence and skill for when the sport comes up at school.

Encouraging little sportsmen and sportswomen

Children are more likely to really put their hearts into their sport if you're their biggest fan. And children who develop a real sporting passion when they're young are more likely to carry on exercising when they grow up – they know how good it feels to be strong and fit, how rewarding it is to see their skills improve and, last but not least, how much fun sports can be!

▶▶ Help them to practise their skills – even if you're dreadful at them yourself.

▶▶ Turn up at as many matches as you can, and cheer like mad!

▶▶ Congratulate them – whether they win, lose or draw.

▶▶ Take them along to professional matches – seeing their sporting heroes in action can be a real inspiration.

Exercise shouldn't take over a child's life – even if they'd like it to (some little sportsmen and women can be incredibly 'driven'!). And be alert for signs that your child might be overdoing things in an attempt to please you. Tell them they don't have to be the world champion – they're great the way they are!

Encourage your child, but don't let them risk 'burn-out'.

Walking with a purpose

Walking is fantastic exercise – it's what human beings were designed for! Other than comfortable shoes, you don't even need any special clothes or equipment.

But what do you do if your child thinks walking is boring? Give your walks a reason, and your child will think they're a treat!

▶▶ Get your child a pedometer – walking is more fun when they can count the steps they take, or the miles they've walked! Vary your routes, so your child can see which one gives the best step and mile total.

▶▶ Make it a nature ramble. Buy, or borrow some field guides from the library, so you can look up the things you saw when you get home. Encourage your child to keep a nature notebook.

▶▶ Get some inexpensive binoculars and go on a birdwatching walk.

▶▶ If you have a regular walk-route, take a camera with you so that you can take pictures of the things you see.

▶▶ Make a 'changes through the year' scrapbook. Each month take photos of certain places on your route, such as 'our front garden', 'the bridge over the river' and 'Jenny's favourite tree'.

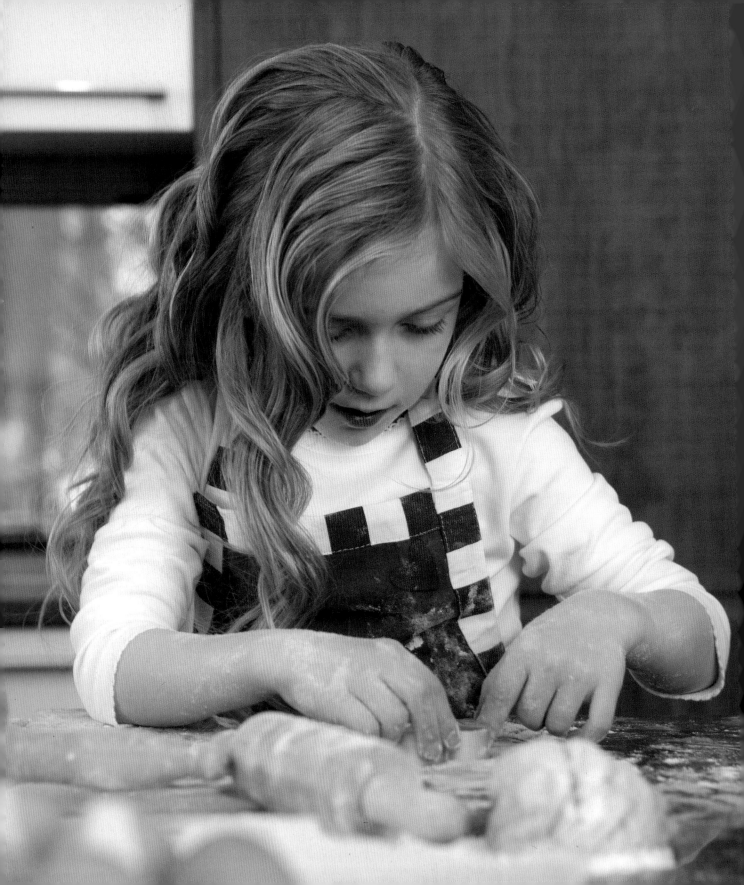

PART 5
RECIPES

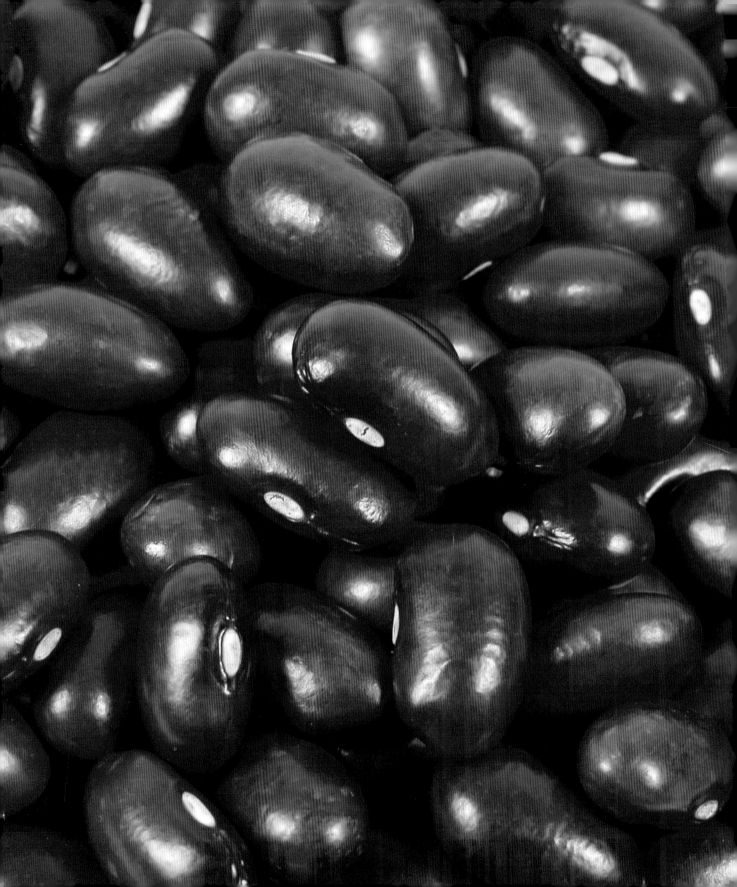

CHAPTER TEN

DELICIOUS JUNK-FREE RECIPES

All of the recipes are simple and adaptable so don't be afraid to experiment. You might like to add additional vegetables to some of the savoury meals or perhaps try different herbs and spices. Get used to tasting food while you are cooking.

All recipes serve 4, unless stated otherwise

KEY TO SYMBOLS

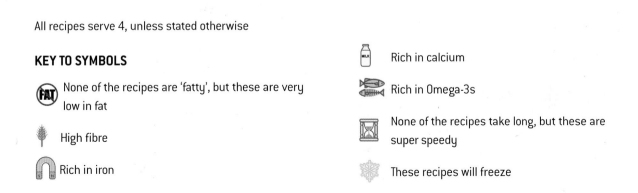

FAT None of the recipes are 'fatty', but these are very low in fat

High fibre

Rich in iron

Rich in calcium

Rich in Omega-3s

None of the recipes take long, but these are super speedy

These recipes will freeze

WEEKEND AND HOLIDAY LUNCH RECIPES

Quick chunky vegetable and pasta soup with a toasted crusty roll

1 large onion, finely chopped

1 clove garlic, crushed (optional)

1 stick of celery, finely diced

1 large carrot, finely diced

1 small leek, finely chopped (optional)

1 small courgette, finely chopped

2 small potatoes, finely chopped

1 small can chopped tomato

1 tbsp tomato purée

1 tsp sugar

750ml vegetable or chicken stock

1 large can cannellini beans, rinsed and drained

50g small pasta shapes (shells or similar)

1 handful of torn basil leaves

Freshly ground black pepper

4 crusty bread rolls

Some grated cheese

1. Lightly oil a large saucepan. Add the onion, garlic and celery and cook gently for 5 minutes without browning. Add the remainder of the vegetables, with the tomatoes, tomato purée, sugar and vegetable stock and simmer for 15 minutes. Add the beans, pasta and basil, and season to taste. Simmer for another 15 minutes and pour into bowls.

2. Split the crusty roll in half and sprinkle over a little grated cheese and place under the grill until the cheese melts. Serve with the soup.

3. You can also serve a small bowl of grated parmesan to sprinkle on the soup at the table.

Tip: Remember, if you are serving soup to children, let it cool a little before putting their bowl on the table. If they burn their mouth, it may put them off soup for years!

Mushroom omelette

(SERVES 1)

8 button mushrooms peeled and sliced

2 medium eggs

1 tbsp water

1 tsp chopped fresh parsley, optional

Salt and pepper

1. Gently stir-fry the mushrooms in a teaspoon of oil in a small frying pan. Remove from the pan.

2. Beat the egg with the water in a bowl. Lightly wipe the pan with olive oil and heat gently. Add the egg mixture and cook until the bottom of the omelette is lightly browned and the top is beginning to set. Add the mushrooms and fold the omelette in half. Cook for a further minute.

3. Serve with three small boiled new potatoes, 2 grilled tomatoes and a small can of sweetcorn.

Variations: Add a slice of cooked ham (fat removed, and chopped) or 25g grated half-fat Cheddar cheese to the omelettes, instead of the mushrooms.

Quick crusty pizza

(SERVES 1)

1 wholemeal roll, split in half

2 tbsp tomato purée

½ tsp dried mixed herbs or tsp fresh chopped parsley (optional)

1 clove garlic, finely sliced

50g low-fat mozzarella cheese, cut into slices

2 tomatoes, sliced

4 mushrooms, sliced

2 slices cooked ham, cut into thin strips

6 olives, sliced (optional)

1. Preheat the oven to 200C/Gas 6.

2. Lay the two halves of the roll – cut side up – on a baking tray.

3. Spread the tomato purée over the halves of the roll, then sprinkle with the herbs. Arrange the tomato slices and mushroom slices over. Sprinkle over the ham, garlic and mozzarella. Sprinkle over the olives, if used.

4. Bake in the oven for 12–15 minutes or until the bread is crisp and the cheese melted and bubbling.

5. Serve immediately with a large green salad.

Variations: Try using other toppings such as onion rings, pineapple and ham and slices of mozzarella or a little grated Cheddar.

Sweet sesame chicken strips with brown rice and salad

160g brown rice

100g frozen peas, cooked

1 small can sweetcorn

2 tbsp runny honey

Juice of one large or 2 small oranges

2 tsp dark soy sauce

1 large clove garlic, finely chopped

1 red pepper, finely chopped

2 tsp olive oil

4 small or 3 large chicken breasts, skinned and thinly sliced

2 tbsp sesame seeds, lightly toasted

1. Cook the rice according to the instructions on the packet. Cook the peas (adding the drained sweetcorn for the last two minutes of cooking time). Drain and keep warm.

2. Combine the honey, orange juice, soy sauce, garlic and red pepper in a bowl. Heat the oil in a non-stick frying pan and fry the chicken strips for two minutes. Add the sauce to the pan and cook, stirring gently for four minutes until the chicken is cooked and coated with a sticky sauce. Add the toasted sesame seeds and stir. Transfer the chicken to a serving dish and keep warm. Combine the peas and sweetcorn with the drained cooked rice and serve.

3. Serve with a mixed salad or green beans.

Chicken dippers with peas and sweetcorn mash, and tomato salsa

4 small chicken breasts, skin removed

1 large egg

100g fine dry breadcrumbs

Freshly ground black pepper

40g parmesan, finely grated (optional)

1. Preheat the oven to 180C/Gas 4.

2. Cut each of the chicken breasts into 2.5cm-wide strips. Beat the egg on a flat plate and put breadcrumbs and ground black pepper (combined with the grated parmesan, if used) on a second plate. Dip the chicken strips into the egg and then into the breadcrumbs to coat thoroughly. Place the chicken strips on a baking tray and spray lightly with a spray oil. Bake the chicken dippers for 15 minutes or until the crumb is golden and the chicken is cooked right through.

To make pea and sweetcorn mash: Boil potatoes and mash with a little milk. Cook a quantity of frozen peas and sweetcorn and drain. Gently stir the drained peas and sweetcorn into the mashed potatoes.

Serve with a good quality bought salsa – check for salt and additives.

To make breadcrumbs: Dry some stale bread in a very low oven until it is crisp but not coloured. Whizz in a blender to make fine breadcrumbs.

Homemade beef burgers

350g lean beef mince

1 small onion, finely chopped

Freshly ground black pepper

40g fresh white breadcrumbs

1 medium egg, beaten

Optional extras – choose from the following:

1 tsp mild mustard

1 tsp creamed horseradish sauce

¼ tsp chilli

1 tbsp tomato sauce

1 tsp Worcestershire sauce

1 clove garlic crushed

1. Place the beef into a bowl. Gently fry the onion in a lightly oiled pan for a couple of minutes until it has softened. Transfer to the bowl. Add freshly ground black pepper, breadcrumbs and one of the optional extras if you like. Add the egg to the bowl and using your hands mix the ingredients together thoroughly. Form into 4 thick burgers. Place on a plate and refrigerate for a short time to allow the burgers to firm up a little.

2. Cook the burgers in a dry frying pan on a gentle heat for 6–8 minutes on each side or until they are cooked through. You can also cook them on a moderate grill for a similar time. Serve in a wholemeal bap, with relish or salsa and a green salad.

Homemade chicken or turkey burgers

350g chicken or turkey, minced

1 medium onion, finely chopped

40g fresh white breadcrumbs

1 clove garlic, crushed

2 tsp soy sauce (optional)

1 medium egg, beaten

1. Combine all of the ingredients in a bowl and mix well. Form into 4 burgers. Place on a plate and refrigerate for a short time to allow the burgers to firm up a little.

2. Lightly oil a frying pan and cook the burgers on a gentle heat for 5–7 minutes on each side or until they are cooked through. You can also cook them on a moderate grill. Serve with a wholemeal bap, slices of cucumber, relish or salsa and a green salad.

Filled jacket potato and salad

(SERVES 1)

🌾 ⧗ if microwaved

A jacket potato with a nutritious topping makes a cheap and simple lunch or supper. If you're short of time, you can cook the potato in the microwave instead of baking, and it will be ready to eat in just a few minutes.

1. Preheat the oven to 200C/Gas 6. Scrub the potato in cold water and dry on kitchen paper. Pierce the potato several times with a fork and bake in the oven for 45 minutes– 1 hour until it's soft. When it's cooked cut a cross in the top of the potato, carefully give it a squeeze to open it up, and pile on the filling.

To microwave: After washing, drying and piercing the potato, place it in the microwave and cook on full power for 2–3 minutes. Turn the potato over and cook for another 2 minutes, or until the potato is soft (the time will depend on the power of your microwave and the size of the potato. If you cook more than one potato in the microwave at a time, you will need to increase the cooking time).

Choose from the following fillings:
▶▶ Reduced-sugar reduced-salt baked beans
▶▶ Low-fat cottage cheese with pineapple, chives, ham or prawn
▶▶ 1 small tin tuna, with sweetcorn and a tablespoon of reduced fat mayonnaise
▶▶ 1 tablespoon of grated half-fat Cheddar cheese with low-fat coleslaw

Chunky potato wedges

(SERVES 2)

(FAT) 🌾

2–3 medium potatoes (together weighing 300g), washed but not peeled
Ground black pepper or Cajun spice or paprika or chilli powder
2 tsp olive oil

1. Preheat the oven to 220C/ Gas 7.

2. Wash the potatoes but leave the skins on. Cut the potatoes in half lengthways, then cut each half lengthways again. Now cut each of the quarters into thick wedges. Put the oil and any seasoning you want to use into a large bowl and add the potatoes. Toss them to get all of the surfaces lightly coated with oil – use your hands, it's messy but easier!

3. Lay the wedges on a non-stick baking tray or non-stick baking paper. Put the wedges into the oven and bake for 25–35 minutes or until the potatoes are tender. Turn them a couple of times during the cooking time so that they brown evenly. Serve immediately.

Wedgie bowls

(ALL SERVE 1)

You could also try one of these for supper on a 'You Choose' day.

1. Put a portion of cooked wedges (150g) in an ovenproof bowl and keep warm. Grill 2 tomato halves and 8 mushroom halves and add to the bowl. Sprinkle over 20g of grated half-fat Cheddar cheese and put under the grill until the cheese melts and bubbles. Serve with a large salad.

2. Put a portion of wedges in an ovenproof bowl and keep warm. Heat a tin of reduced-sugar, reduced-salt baked beans in the microwave until piping hot. Add to the wedges in the bowl. Sprinkle over 20g of grated half-fat Cheddar cheese and grill until the cheese melts and bubbles. Serve with a large salad.

3. Put a portion of wedges into an ovenproof bowl and keep warm. Cut two slices of lean ham into bite sized pieces and pile over the wedges. Top with 20g grated half-fat Cheddar cheese and grill until the cheese melts and bubbles. Serve with a large salad.

4. Put a portion of potato wedges in a bowl. Top with two tablespoons of baked beans (heated), and a grilled, sliced vegetarian or low-fat sausage. Serve with a small salad.

5. Top a portion of potato wedges with a slice of ham or chicken (shredded), sweetcorn, and a sprinkling of grated cheese.

Pronto pasta and sauce

(FAT) 🌾 if wholemeal pasta ⧗

300g pasta shapes

1 red pepper, deseeded and diced

1 green pepper, deseeded and diced

1 red onion, finely chopped

1 quantity of basic tomato sauce (below)

Handful of basil leaves, roughly torn (optional)

For the basic tomato sauce:

1 tsp olive oil

1 medium onion finely chopped

1 clove garlic finely chopped

1 can chopped tomatoes

1 tbsp tomato purée

1 tsp sugar

Freshly ground black pepper

To make the basic tomato sauce: Put the olive oil into a large saucepan and gently fry the onions and garlic until softened but not coloured. Add the other ingredients, stir to combine. Place a lid on the saucepan and simmer the sauce gently for 15 minutes.

Variations: This basic tomato sauce can be used as a base for stews and casseroles and for a variety of pasta sauces. You can add other vegetables such as broccoli, sweetcorn, peppers, peas, spring onions or courgette to the sauce. It can also be used as a base for mince, soya or Quorn mince dishes.

1. Serve with the pasta, and a large salad.

DINNER RECIPES
CHICKEN (OR TURKEY) DAYS

Sticky chicken with fresh boiled vegetables and mash

4 small boneless chicken breasts, skinned

1 tbsp sweet pickle or mango chutney

1 tsp olive oil

1 tsp honey

1 tsp tomato purée (optional)

2 tbsp water

1. Preheat the oven to 180C/Gas 4.

2. Place the chicken breasts on a large piece of foil. Combine the other ingredients in a small bowl and spoon over the breasts. Loosely wrap the foil around the chicken to make a parcel. Bake in the oven for 25–30 minutes, or until the chicken is thoroughly cooked. Uncover the chicken for the final 10 minutes of cooking time.

3. Slice each of the breasts into 4–6 slices and arrange on individual plates. You could place the meat on small mounds of baby salad leaves to serve.

4. Serve with mashed or boiled potatoes and fresh vegetables.

Speedy chicken and vegetable stir-fry with brown rice or noodles

1 tsp vegetable oil

4 small chicken breasts, skin removed and thinly sliced

1 small onion, finely sliced

1 clove garlic, finely chopped

16 small broccoli florets

12 medium mushrooms, sliced

200g beansprouts

1 red pepper, deseeded and sliced

½ green pepper

2 tbsp water

1 tbsp light soy sauce

1 tsp honey (optional)

1. Heat the oil in a wok or large frying pan and cook the chicken until it is cooked right through. Remove on to a plate. Put the onion and garlic into the pan and stir-fry for 3 minutes. Add the remaining vegetables and fry for 2 minutes stirring all the time. Add the water and cook for a further minute.

2. Add the cooked chicken, soy sauce and honey and cook for 1–2 minutes until the chicken is piping hot. Serve on a bed of brown rice or noodles.

Muffin chicken pizza with salad

1 small tin chopped tomatoes

2 tsp tomato purée

½ tsp sugar, optional

½ tsp mixed herbs (if liked)

4 wholemeal English muffins, split in half

8 mushrooms, thinly sliced

4 tbsp sweetcorn (if liked)

8 slices of cold cooked chicken (not processed slices)

2 tomatoes, sliced

3 tbsp grated Cheddar or 60g mozzarella cheese, sliced

1. Heat the oven to 180C/Gas Mark 4.

2. Place the tinned tomatoes in a saucepan. Boil gently until they have reduced to a thick sauce. Add the tomato purée, sugar and herbs if liked. Allow to cool slightly.

3. Lightly toast the eight halves of muffin and top with the cooled tomato mixture, the mushroom slices, sweetcorn, chicken (cut into small pieces) and tomato slices. Sprinkle over the cheese.

4. Bake for 10–12 minutes until the muffins are crisp and the cheese is melted. Serve with a large salad.

Baked chicken breast with sweetcorn mash and fresh boiled vegetables

4 small chicken breasts, skinned

Freshly ground black pepper or Cajun seasoning

300g mashed potato

1 small tin sweetcorn

1. Preheat the oven to 180C/Gas Mark 4.

2. Place the chicken breasts on a piece of baking foil, sprinkle with black pepper or Cajun seasoning. Wrap into a loose parcel and bake in the oven for 25–30 minutes or until the chicken is cooked right through.

3. Boil and mash the potatoes, adding a little milk if desired. Drain and rinse the sweetcorn. Heat the sweetcorn in a small saucepan with a little water. Drain when hot and add to the mashed potatoes. Pile the mashed potatoes into a serving dish and place under the grill until the potatoes are lightly golden.

4. Slice the chicken. Serve with the sweetcorn mash and fresh boiled vegetables – peas or French beans are ideal.

5. Children may like a tomato sauce to dip their chicken into. Just combine a little low-sugar tomato ketchup with an equal quantity of water in a small bowl.

This is a great way to cook chicken if you want 'roast' chicken for Sunday lunch and don't want to cook a whole chicken. All you need to do is slice it when it is cooked, and make a gravy.

Spanish chicken with pasta and green salad

4 small chicken breasts, skinned

1 medium onion, sliced

2 small green peppers, deseeded and sliced

1 clove garlic, crushed

1 tbsp fresh basil, chopped (optional)

Large tin chopped tomatoes

$\frac{1}{2}$ tsp dried oregano or mixed herbs

8 green or black olives, stoned (optional)

Ground black pepper

150ml chicken stock

1. Fry the chicken breast in a non-stick pan wiped with oil, to seal. Add the onions and pepper and cook for 5 minutes. Add the garlic, herbs, tinned tomatoes, dried herbs, olives, black pepper and stock. Reduce heat, place a lid on the pan and simmer gently for 20 minutes until the chicken is tender. (Check once or twice to see that the liquid has not evaporated and add a little water or stock if necessary.)

2. Spoon into a serving dish and sprinkle over the basil, if used. Serve with a portion of penne pasta or spaghetti and a green salad or green beans and broccoli.

Turkey burger with chunky chips and green salad

200g lean turkey mince

1 small onion, peeled and very finely chopped

1 medium carrot, grated

1 tbsp tomato purée

Freshly ground black pepper

1 tbsp fresh parsley, finely chopped (optional)

1. Put all of the ingredients into a bowl and mix together thoroughly. Form into 4 burgers. Grill or cook gently in a dry non-stick pan for 6–8 minutes on each side until they are golden and completely cooked through.

2. Serve with a portion of Homemade Chunky Chips (see page 141) and a green salad. Or you could have a toasted burger bap instead of the Chunky Chips. If you use a burger bap, add some lettuce, cucumber and tomato slices to the roll and sit the burger on top of them.

FISH DAYS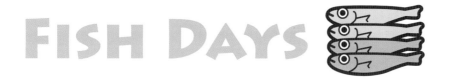

Pan-cooked cod or haddock fillet with homemade chunky chips, grilled tomatoes, peas or broccoli

(FAT)

4 fillets of cod or haddock

Flour to coat the fish

Freshly ground black pepper

1. Dust the fish on both sides with a little flour and sprinkle with freshly ground black pepper.

2. Spray a non-stick frying pan with a little light spray oil (olive oil in a spray can) and gently pan-cook the fish until it is golden and cooked through, turning once.

3. Serve with chunky chips, grilled tomatoes and peas or broccoli.

For the Chunky Chips:

4–6 medium potatoes (together weighing 300g)

4 tsp oil

Freshly ground pepper, if liked

1. Preheat oven to 220C/ Gas 7.

2. Wash the potatoes but don't peel them. Cut into chunky chips. Boil the potatoes for 3 minutes then drain and cool immediately under cold water. Place the oil in a bowl and add the chips. Toss to lightly coat them in the oil – use your hands, it's easier. Lay the chips on a non-stick baking tray or a piece of non-stick baking paper. Bake for 25–35 minutes until they are cooked and golden. Turn a couple of times during cooking so that the chips brown evenly. If they brown too quickly turn the oven heat down a little.

Grilled or pan-fried fresh salmon with boiled new potatoes and vegetables

4 salmon fillets

Sweet chilli dipping sauce (if liked)

1. Spray a non-stick frying pan with a little light spray oil (olive oil in a spray can) and gently pan-fry the fish until it is cooked, turning once.

2. Transfer the fish to a plate and drizzle over a teaspoon of sweet chilli dipping sauce if liked.

3. Serve with boiled new potatoes, and a selection of fresh boiled or steamed vegetables.

Homemade fish fingers with chunky chips, peas and grilled tomatoes

450g cod, haddock or other firm white fish

1 medium egg, beaten

50g fine wholemeal breadcrumbs

25g oat flakes or finely crushed cornflakes

Spray vegetable oil to fry or bake

Salt and pepper

1. Check carefully to ensure that no bones have been left in the fish, then slice the fillets into 'fish finger'-sized slices. Pour the beaten egg into a shallow dish and put the mixed crumbs on to a plate. Dip the fish pieces into the egg and then into the crumb. Spray some vegetable oil into a non-stick frying pan and fry gently until the fish fingers are golden on both sides. Drain on kitchen towel and serve with homemade chunky chips, peas and grilled tomatoes or broccoli. Serve with homemade chunky chips (page 141).

You can also bake the fish fingers if you prefer. Preheat the oven to 180C/Gas 4. Place the fish on a baking tray covered with a piece of non-stick baking parchment. Spray with a little oil and bake for 12–15 minutes until the fish is cooked.

Remember, do not freeze homemade fish fingers unless you are sure that the fish has not already been frozen and defrosted.

Baked cod with breadcrumb topping, mashed potatoes and a selection of vegetables or green salad

4 fillets of fresh cod (or frozen cod, defrosted)

3 slices wholemeal bread, made into crumbs

4 tsp Cheddar cheese, grated

Freshly ground black pepper

1 tbsp parsley (optional)

2 tsp olive oil

1. Preheat the oven to 180C/Gas 4.

2. Place the fillets on a non-stick baking tray. Place the breadcrumbs in a small bowl. Add all of the other ingredients to the bowl and mix together. Press on to the top of the fillets and bake in the oven for 12–15 minutes or until the fish is cooked through (this will depend on the thickness of the fish) and the topping is crisp.

3. Serve with mashed (or boiled potatoes) and a selection of fresh vegetables or salad.

Speedy tuna or salmon and tomato pasta with salad

and if salmon used.

200g pasta shapes (penne, bows, shells etc)

2 small cans tuna in brine, or salmon, drained

2 tbsp tomato purée

1 tbsp olive oil

1 clove garlic, peeled and crushed (if liked)

1 large can tomatoes, chopped

Freshly ground black pepper

1. Cook the pasta according to the packet instructions, then drain.

2. Combine all of the other ingredients in a large saucepan. Heat gently until hot. Stir in the pasta and heat for a further minute.

3. Serve with a large green salad.

Prawn and vegetable stir-fry with noodles or rice

300g bag ready prepared stir-fry vegetables with a sachet
  of stir-fry sauce
2 tbsp water
200g frozen prawns, defrosted
2 tsp soy sauce
Freshly ground black pepper

1. Lightly oil a non-stick pan and fry the vegetables as instructed on the packaging. Stir in the prawns and sauce and heat through. Do not overcook the prawns or they will be tough.

2. Serve with wholemeal rice or noodles and a large mixed salad.

BEAN DAYS

Spicy lentil casserole with brown rice or boiled new potatoes and fresh vegetables or salad

1 medium onion, chopped
150g mushrooms, quartered
1 large can tomatoes, chopped
1 small courgette, diced
1 large green or red pepper, deseeded and diced
150ml water or stock
A pinch of chilli powder or paprika (optional)
2 cans green or Continental lentils
2 tbsp natural low-fat yoghurt (optional)
1 tbsp chopped fresh coriander (optional)

1. Lightly oil a large saucepan and fry the onion until softened. Add the mushrooms, tomatoes, courgette and pepper, and the water or stock. Add the paprika or chilli powder, if used. Bring to the boil, lower the heat and simmer for 10 minutes. Drain and rinse the lentils and add to the saucepan. Simmer gently for another 5 minutes. Turn into a dish, add the tablespoon of natural yoghurt and the fresh coriander if used.

2. Serve with potatoes or brown rice and a green salad or fresh vegetables.

Chickpea and vegetable chilli with brown rice and a green salad or fresh boiled vegetables

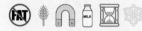

1 medium onion, chopped

1 small clove garlic, crushed

1 large can tomatoes

$1/4$ tsp chilli powder (or to taste)

150ml vegetable stock

$1/2$ tsp sugar

1 large can of chickpeas, rinsed and drained

2 medium carrots, chopped

10 cauliflower florets

1 red pepper, deseeded and chopped

10 broccoli florets

1 tbsp low-fat natural yoghurt (optional)

1. Lightly oil a saucepan and fry the onion until softened. Add the garlic, tomatoes and spices and cook for a further minute. Add the stock and sugar. Add the chickpeas and other vegetables and simmer until the vegetables are just tender (about 8 minutes). Just before serving stir in the yoghurt, if used.

2. Serve with brown rice and a green salad or fresh vegetables

Spicy bean fajita wraps with a green salad

1 medium onion, peeled and chopped

1 red pepper, deseeded, quartered and cut into strips

1 clove garlic crushed (if liked)

Pinch of Cajun seasoning, chilli powder or $1/2$ tsp fajita seasoning

1 can red kidney beans or pinto beans, rinsed and drained

1 large can chopped tomatoes

50g grated half-fat cheddar cheese

4 soft wheat or corn tortillas

1. Preheat the oven to 180C/Gas 4.

2. Spray a saucepan with a little olive oil spray, and gently fry the onion, pepper and garlic for 3 minutes. Add the spice, beans and half of the chopped tomatoes and cook gently for 5 minutes until the sauce has thickened a little.

3. Spread some of the mixture on to each of the tortillas and roll up. Place them seam side down in an ovenproof dish. Spoon over the remaining tomato and sprinkle the cheese over.

4. Bake for 10–15 minutes until the cheese is melted and golden.

5. Serve with a large salad.

Oven-baked bean burgers with a wholemeal bap and salad

1 large tin red kidney beans

1 can cannellini beans

1 small onion, finely chopped

1 clove garlic, crushed (optional)

1/2 red pepper, finely chopped

1 medium carrot, finely grated

1/4 tsp ground cumin

1/4 tsp ground coriander

Freshly ground black pepper

1 tbsp tomato purée

4 tbsp fresh wholemeal breadcrumbs

1 small egg, beaten

1. Drain, rinse and mash the beans in a large bowl. Lightly fry the onion, garlic and red pepper in an oiled frying pan until it has softened and then add the spices and cook for a further 2 minutes. Add to the mashed beans and mix together. Add the tomato purée and the breadcrumbs and enough egg to bind the mixture together. Form into 4 burgers.

2. Add a little oil to a non-stick pan and cook the burgers for 5–8 minutes on each side until they are crisp and golden.

3. You can also bake the burgers if you prefer. Heat the oven to 180C/Gas 4. Place the burgers on to non-stick baking parchment and spray with a little oil. Bake in the oven for 20–25 minutes until crisp and golden. Turn the burgers once during the cooking time.

4. Split a wholemeal bap and add a tablespoon of pickle (choose a low-sugar brand), cucumber slices and tomato slices. Place the burger on top, and top with the other half of the bap. Serve with a large salad.

5. Why not make a batch of bean burgers and freeze to use later? Children will love helping to make them.

Beany braise with fresh steamed vegetables

1 onion, finely chopped

1 red or green pepper, deseeded and finely chopped

1 large can chopped tomatoes

1 tbsp tomato purée

3 tbsp water

Freshly ground black pepper

1 can haricot beans, rinsed and drained

1 can cannellini beans, rinsed and drained

2 bread rolls torn into chunks

2 tbsp grated cheese

1. Pre-heat the oven to 160C/Gas 3.

2. Gently fry the chopped onion and the pepper for 2–3 minutes until softened. Add the chopped tomato, tomato purée, water and ground black pepper and simmer for 5 minutes. Add the drained beans and cook for a further 10 minutes on a low heat. Transfer to an ovenproof dish and sprinkle over the torn pieces of roll. Sprinkle over the grated cheese. Place in the preheated oven and bake for 10–15 minutes until the cheese has melted and the bread is crisp.

3. Serve with fresh steamed or boiled vegetables.

French bean stew with crusty bread

2 tsp olive oil

2 medium onions, thinly sliced

1 clove garlic, crushed

2 sticks celery, sliced (optional)

1 large red pepper, deseeded and sliced

1 large green pepper, deseeded and sliced

1 can chopped tomatoes

2 tbsp tomato purée

1 tsp sugar

150ml water

1 tsp dried thyme

1 bay leaf

1 can pinto or cannellini beans, rinsed and drained

8 black olives, sliced (optional)

A handful of torn basil leaves

1. Heat 2 teaspoons of oil in a large saucepan and gently fry the onion, garlic and celery if used for 5 minutes. Add the peppers and fry for a further 5 minutes, stirring frequently. Add the can of tomatoes, the tomato purée, sugar, water, thyme and bay leaf and cook for a further 10 minutes. Add the washed and drained beans and cook for another 10 minutes. Stir in the basil leaves.

2. Serve with broccoli and green beans and some warmed crusty bread.

VEGETARIAN DAYS

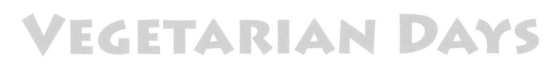

Cowboy 'sausage' and beans with mashed (or jacket) potato and broccoli

4 Quorn or vegetarian sausages

1 medium onion, peeled and chopped

4 large tomatoes, peeled and chopped

1 large tin and 1 small tin reduced-sugar and reduced-salt
baked beans

Pinch of chilli or paprika (more if you like it) or 1 tsp
Worcestershire sauce (optional)

3 tbsp water or stock

1. Gently fry (in a non-stick pan wiped with oil) or grill the sausages until they are browned and cooked through. Cut into pieces.

2. Spray a small amount of oil into a non-stick saucepan and gently fry the onion for 2 minutes, add the tomato and fry for a couple more minutes until the onions and tomato are soft. Add the beans and the cooked sausage pieces. Stir and heat until piping hot. Stir in the spice or Worcestershire sauce if liked.

3. Serve with mashed potato or a small jacket potato and broccoli or green beans.

Veggie frittata with salad and a wholemeal bap or boiled new potatoes

5 medium eggs, beaten

2 tbsp water

Ground black pepper

$\frac{1}{4}$ tsp mixed herbs (optional)

Spray oil for pan

$\frac{1}{2}$ medium onion, finely sliced

1 red pepper, deseeded and finely diced

10 small mushrooms, quartered

1 small can sweetcorn, drained

150g cooked new potatoes cut into small dice

1. In a small bowl beat the eggs with the water, black pepper and mixed herbs if used; set aside. Spray a medium-sized non-stick frying pan with a little oil and fry the onions, pepper and mushrooms for a few minutes until they are softened. Add the sweetcorn and diced potatoes to the pan and pour over the egg mixture.

2. Cook gently for about 6–8 minutes until the egg begins to set. Place under a grill to brown and set the top. Cut the frittata into wedges and serve with a green salad and a warmed wholemeal bap.

Egg and mushroom pan-fry with vegetables and a wholemeal bap

1 tsp olive oil

1 small onion, finely chopped

200g button mushrooms, wiped and thinly sliced

5 medium eggs, beaten

2 tbsp milk

1 tbsp fresh parsley, chopped

Freshly ground black pepper

10 cherry tomatoes, halved

40g half-fat Cheddar cheese, grated

1. Lightly oil a medium-sized non-stick frying pan and fry the onion and mushrooms gently for 2 minutes. Beat the eggs in a small bowl with the milk and parsley. Season to taste. Add the egg mixture to the mushrooms and onion in the pan and stir over a low heat until the eggs are lightly set. Arrange the cherry tomato halves on top of the egg and sprinkle with the cheese. Place under a hot grill until the cheese is melted and golden, and the egg is completely set. Cut the pan-fry into wedges and serve with boiled fresh vegetables and a wholemeal bap or new potatoes.

Broccoli, cauliflower and sweetcorn cheese with boiled new potatoes and grilled tomatoes

200g broccoli florets

200g cauliflower florets

1 small can sweetcorn, drained

50g butter or low-fat spread

½ pint semi-skimmed milk

50g flour

75g Cheddar cheese grated

A few drops of Worcestershire sauce, if liked

Freshly ground black pepper

For the crispy topping (optional):

1 slice bread, crumbed

1 tbsp grated cheese

1. Cook the broccoli and cauliflower florets until tender, adding the drained sweetcorn for the last 2 minutes. Drain. Meanwhile make the cheese sauce by melting the butter or low-fat spread in a saucepan, adding the flour, then gradually adding the milk and beating until smooth. Bring to the boil, stirring all the time. Add the grated Cheddar cheese and continue stirring until the cheese has melted. Arrange the vegetables in a dish and pour over the sauce.

2. For a crisp topping, combine the breadcrumbs and cheese and sprinkle over the dish. Grill until the cheese has melted and the breadcrumbs are golden.

Vegetarian sausage topper, with baked beans, grilled tomatoes, jacket potato and salad and low-fat coleslaw

4 medium (150g) jacket potatoes

4 Quorn (or vegetarian) sausages

4 medium tomatoes, halved

1 large can baked beans

4 tbsp low-fat coleslaw (optional)

1. Cook the jacket potatoes in the oven or microwave and keep warm. Fry the sausages in a dry non-stick frying pan, or grill them. Grill the tomato halves and heat the baked beans. Cut the sausages into pieces and mix with the beans.

2. Split the potatoes and pile the beans and sausage mixture on the top. Serve with the grilled tomato and the low-fat coleslaw (if liked) and salad.

Mild egg and vegetable curry with rice

1 large onion, finely chopped

1 eating apple, peeled and finely chopped

1 clove garlic, crushed or finely chopped

150 ml water or vegetable stock

½ can 'light' coconut milk

200g green beans, each cut into three pieces

16 small cauliflower florets

3 tomatoes cut into wedges

150g frozen peas

2 tbsp sultanas

4 eggs

2 tsp mild curry powder, or to taste

1. Lightly oil a large non-stick saucepan and gently fry the chopped onions, apple and garlic for 5 minutes until they have softened. Add the curry powder, cook for a minute more. Add the water, coconut milk, green beans and cauliflower. Cover the pan and simmer for 8–10 minutes until the beans and cauliflower are cooked (you may need to add a little more water). Add the tomato wedges, the frozen peas and the sultanas, if used, and cook for another 3 minutes.

2. Meanwhile, place the eggs in a saucepan of water and boil for 10 minutes. Remove from the heat and cool under running cold water immediately. Remove the eggshells and cut each egg in half lengthways. Lay the eggs cut side down in the bottom of a shallow dish.

3. When the curry sauce is ready pour it over the halved eggs and serve with brown or white rice and a green salad.

'You Choose' Days

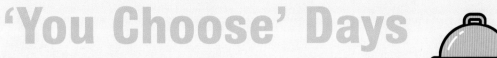

Here are a few more recipes you might like to try on a 'You Choose Day'

Roasted lamb steaks with mashed or boiled new potatoes and green vegetables

4 small lamb leg steaks, all fat and skin removed

1 medium onion, finely sliced, lengthways

1 tbsp runny honey

2 tbsp red wine vinegar or water

2 tbsp mint, washed and finely chopped

Freshly ground black pepper

1. Preheat the oven to 200C/Gas 6.

2. Lay the lamb steaks in a shallow ovenproof dish. Combine the onion, honey, vinegar or water, mint and black pepper. Pour the marinade over the steaks. Turn the steaks to coat both sides in the marinade. Bake the steaks for 15–20 minutes until they are cooked. Baste the steaks with the marinade once or twice during the cooking time. Place on a warm serving dish and spoon over any remaining marinade.

3. Serve with mashed or boiled new potatoes and green vegetables.

Sweet and simple pork with vegetable rice

4 lean pork chops, all skin and fat removed

2 tbsp tomato purée

1 tsp lemon juice

1tbsp water

1 tbsp runny honey

1 tbsp Worcestershire sauce

Freshly ground black pepper

160g brown rice

250g cooked frozen mixed vegetables

1. Lay the pork chops on foil on a grill pan. Combine the tomato purée, lemon juice, water, honey, Worcestershire sauce and pepper in a small bowl and brush on to both sides of the chops. Grill for 15 minutes, turning frequently and brushing with the sauce, until the meat is cooked and well glazed. Transfer to a warmed serving plate.

2. Meanwhile, cook the rice according to the packet instructions and combine with the vegetables.

Stir-fried beef with noodles and steamed broccoli

300g lean rump steak, fat removed and cut into strips

1 tbsp soy sauce

5 tbsp water

1 tbsp cornflour

2 tsp vegetable oil

6 spring onions cut into 3cm-long pieces

300g ready-prepared stir-fry vegetables

100g mushrooms, thinly sliced

1 clove garlic, finely chopped

½ tsp Chinese 5 spice powder (optional)

1. Place the strips of beef into a bowl with 1 teaspoon of the soy sauce, 1 tablespoon of water and the cornflour and mix together. Heat 1 teaspoon of the oil in a large frying pan or wok and stir-fry the beef for 2–3 minutes over a high heat. Remove the meat from the pan with a slotted spoon and set aside.

2. Place the remaining teaspoon of oil into the pan and stir-fry the vegetables and mushrooms for 3–4 minutes. Add the remaining water, the Chinese 5 spice powder (if used) and the remaining soy sauce. Return the beef to the pan and cook for a further 2 minutes.

3. Serve with noodles or rice and steamed broccoli (or Chinese greens).

The secret of speedy stir-fry cooking is to get all of the ingredients ready before starting to cook. Then it really is quick.

DESSERT RECIPES

Plum and almond crumble

500g plums, washed, halved and stones removed

1 tablespoon light brown sugar

125g plain wholemeal flour

50g soft brown sugar

50g butter, cut into cubes

50g ground almonds

1. Preheat the oven to 180C/Gas 4.

2. Arrange the prepared plums in a deep ovenproof dish. Place the flour, sugar and cubes of butter into a bowl and rub in the fat until the mixture resembles breadcrumbs. Stir in the ground almonds. Spoon the crumble mixture evenly over the plums and press down lightly.

3. Bake in the oven for 40–45 minutes until the plums are cooked and the crumble is golden. Serve with custard made with skimmed milk, or low-fat natural yoghurt.

4. The crumble topping can be used to make a variety of other fruit crumbles. Why not try: apples, apricots, apple and blackberries or apple and raspberry.

Baked bananas

3 tbsp orange juice

4 tbsp sultanas

1 tsp soft brown sugar

4 small bananas

1. Preheat the oven to 180C/Gas 4.

2. Combine the orange juice, sultanas and brown sugar in a small bowl. Place each of the bananas on a square of foil and spoon over the mixture. Wrap the bananas loosely in the foil to enclose them. Place the bananas in their foil parcels on a baking tray and bake for 15 minutes. Serve with a couple of tablespoons of natural yoghurt.

Strawberry meringue delight

500g carton low-fat fromage frais

2 tbsp lemon or orange curd

3 meringue nests, broken into pieces

250g fresh strawberries, hulled washed and sliced

1. Place the fromage frais in a large bowl and stir in the lemon or orange curd. Gently mix in the broken pieces of the meringue nests. Reserve 8 of the strawberry slices and share the remainder among 4 tall glasses or bowls. Spoon over the fromage frais mixture and decorate the top with the reserved strawberry slices.

Scotch pancake stack with berry fruits and quark

110g self-raising flour (white or wholemeal)

25g caster or soft brown sugar

1 medium egg, beaten

3 tbsp milk

A little oil

Fruit, fromage frais, yoghurt or Quark to serve

1. Sift the flour into a bowl and add the sugar. Thoroughly whisk in the beaten egg and the milk, until you have a smooth, thick batter.

2. Heat a heavy-based non-stick frying pan or griddle and lightly wipe with oil. Drop separate tablespoons of batter into the pan and cook until bubbles rise on the top of the pancakes. Turn over and cook the other side of the pancake until it is golden.

3. Loosely wrap the pancakes in a clean tea towel to keep warm while you cook the rest.

4. Serve a stack of three pancakes with a handful of berries, or slices of a sweet fruit, and a tablespoon of fromage frais or Quark. (You can use stewed fruit or, if you are short of time, try drained tinned or cartons of fruit which has been canned in juice not syrup.)

5. These freeze well so it's worth making a double quantity. Cook, allow to get cold and freeze interleaved with cling film or circles of non-stick baking parchment.

Orangey pears with fromage frais

4 tbsp thin cut marmalade

Small carton of fresh orange juice

4 small pears, peeled

Natural low-fat fromage frais to serve

1. Place the marmalade and the orange juice in a small saucepan and heat over a low heat until the marmalade has melted. Add the whole pears, cover the pan and cook on a low heat for about 10 minutes or until the pears are tender.

2. Serve with the fromage frais.

SPECIAL RECIPES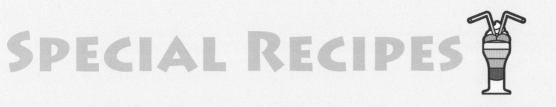

make your own muesli

Get the children to help you make your own special 'family muesli' packed full of the things you all like. When buying cereal to include in your muesli, remember to look for those that aren't loaded with sugar. Look for those with no added sugars, or at least with sugars way down the ingredients list.

Basic recipe

Cereals: 175g rolled oats made up to 250g with any from the Cereals list below

Seeds: 25g made up of any from the Seeds list

Nuts: 25g made up of any from the Nuts list, chopped

Dried fruit: 150g made up of any from the Dried fruits list, chopped if large

1 tsp cinnamon (optional)

Cereals:

wheat bran

bran flakes or sticks

millet flakes

rice flakes

Seeds:

sesame

sunflower

pumpkin

linseeds

Nuts:

toasted hazelnuts

almonds

brazil nuts

cashew nuts

walnuts

pecan nuts

Dried fruits:

sultanas

raisins

ready-to-eat dried apricots, prunes, banana, pear, peach

This will make 12–14 servings. Store in an airtight container. Make small quantities of muesli at a time so that it is fresh, and you will be able to change the ingredients.

Quick banana smoothie

(SERVES 2)

1 large ripe banana

1 small carton natural yogurt

1 tsp honey

100 ml milk

1. Blend all of the ingredients together until smooth. Pour into two glasses.

Nectarine and banana milk shake

(SERVES 1)

1 nectarine, peeled and stoned

1 small banana, sliced

1 small carton natural yogurt

150 ml skimmed milk, chilled

1. Purée the fruit in a blender. Add the yoghurt and milk and blend until frothy. Pour into a glass and serve.

Fast fruity muffins

(MAKES 12 MUFFINS)

125g wholemeal self-raising flour

125g white self-raising flour

30g soft brown sugar

Pinch of salt

2 tbsp vegetable oil

200ml semi-skimmed or skimmed milk

1 medium egg, beaten

75g dried fruit (sultanas, raisins or dried cranberries)

1. Preheat the oven to 220C/Gas 7.

2. Combine the flour and salt in a bowl with the sugar. Add the oil, milk and beaten egg. Stir in the dried fruit. Mix together lightly – the secret of light muffins is not to over-mix.

3. Place 12 cake cases into a muffin tray and spoon the mixture into the cases. Bake for 15 minutes until they are well risen and golden.

Fruity bar

(MAKES 18 FINGERS)

This is great for a lunchbox treat and is high in energy.
(Choose no more than twice a week.)

75g low-fat spread

3 tbsp honey

2 tbsp water

150g porridge oats

½ tsp cinnamon

50g almonds, roughly chopped

50g sunflower seeds

75g raisins or sultanas

8 ready to eat dried apricots, roughly chopped

4 prunes or dates, roughly chopped

20g sesame seeds

1. Preheat the oven 190C/Gas 5.

2. Melt the low-fat spread, honey and water in a large
saucepan over a low heat. Cook for 3 minutes, stirring
continuously (it should thicken slightly).

3. Add all the remaining ingredients and stir thoroughly.
Line a 30cm x 19cm Swiss roll tin with non-stick baking
parchment. Spoon the mixture into the tin and flatten the
surface.

4. Bake for 25–30 minutes until the mixture is firm and a
light golden colour. Remove from the oven and leave to cool
for 10 minutes. Mark into 18 small fingers (divide the tin into
2 along the short edge and 9 along the long edge) and allow
to cool completely. When the bar is cold cut along the marks.
Store the fingers in an airtight tin.

Muesli squares

Another lunchbox favourite.

60g runny honey

50g soft brown sugar

125g butter or low-fat spread suitable for cooking

2 large or 3 medium bananas, mashed

300g muesli (unsweetened)

160g chopped prunes

50g sunflower or pumpkin seeds

1 tsp ground cinnamon

Zest and juice of an orange

1. Preheat the oven to 180C/Gas 4 and line or lightly grease
a 33 x 25 cm shallow non-stick baking tin.

2. Place the muesli and spices in a bowl. Melt the honey,
sugar and butter or low-fat spread in a saucepan over a low
heat. Mash the bananas and add to the muesli, with the
prunes, and the pumpkin seeds. Add the melted mixture to
the dry ingredients with the orange juice and zest. Mix well
together and press into the baking tin. Bake for 25–30
minutes or until golden. Leave to cool in the tin then cut into
small squares or fingers.

Oat jack fingers

60g self-raising wholemeal flour

80g porridge oats

1 tsp mixed spice

40g soft brown sugar

Zest and juice of 1 medium orange

80g ready-to-eat apricots, chopped

40g sultanas

115g butter or low-fat spread suitable for cooking

1 tbsp golden syrup

1. Preheat the oven to 180C/Gas 4.

2. Lightly grease or line a square 18cm x 18cm low-sided baking tray.

3. Combine the flour, oats, spice and sugar in a mixing bowl. Place the orange juice, zest, apricots and sultanas in a small saucepan and simmer gently until the orange juice is absorbed. Leave to cool.

4. Place the margarine and the golden syrup in a small saucepan and heat gently until the margarine has melted. Cool slightly and pour on to the dry ingredients, add the cooled fruit mixture and stir together well.

5. Press into the baking tray and bake on the middle shelf for 25–30 minutes until golden. Take out of the oven, allow to cool for 10 minutes and then mark into small fingers. Leave to cool completely in the tin – this prevents the pieces from breaking when you take them out. Store in an airtight container.

Pancakes

(MAKES AROUND 8 PANCAKES)

This is a simple basic pancake mix which you can use with a variety of fillings. Pancakes can be frozen after they have been cooked and allowed to get cold. If you're short of time you can always use ready-made pancakes from the supermarket. Look for ones that don't contain hydrogenated vegetable oil.

150g plain flour

1 tsp sugar

3 medium eggs, beaten

250ml semi-skimmed milk

A little spray oil for frying

1. Sift the flour into a large bowl. Add the sugar. Make a well in the centre and add the eggs. Beat thoroughly and then gradually add the milk to make a thin smooth batter.

2. Lightly spray a non-stick frying pan and add 3 tablespoons of the batter to the pan. Tilt the pan so that the batter completely covers the surface. Cook until bubbles appear all over the pancake, then turn to cook the other side. Keep the pancake warm until you have cooked as many as you need.

Here are some ideas for sweet fillings:

▶▶ Lemon or orange juice and a sprinkling of sugar

▶▶ Stewed fruit

▶▶ Apple purée

▶▶ Raspberries, strawberries or blueberries mixed with a little low-fat fromage frais

▶▶ A couple of squares of good quality chocolate chopped and mixed with low-fat fromage frais

Granola

This is an ideal crunchy snack — just put a little in a small plastic container or zip-lock bag — or with milk as a breakfast cereal. You can make it with whatever you have in the store cupboard. It's also a tasty topping for desserts.

40g nuts (walnuts, hazelnuts, Brazil nuts, almonds)
350g jumbo oats
25g wheatgerm
2 tbsp sunflower oil
1 tbsp runny honey
50g pumpkin seeds
50g sunflower seeds
25g sesame seeds

1. Preheat the oven to 180C/Gas 4.

2. Chop the nuts and mix with the oats and wheatgerm in a large bowl. Gently warm the oil and the honey. Add to the dry mixture and mix well.

3. Lay the granola on to a large shallow baking tray and bake for about half an hour until it is lightly browned. Turn the mixture once or twice and if it appears to be browning too quickly lower the oven heat.

4. Allow to cool completely and store in an airtight container.

INDEX